高等教育出版社 中国·北京
Higher Education Press, Beijing, China

英漢實用中醫藥大全

趙樸初題

7

OPHTHALMOLOGY
眼科學

THE ENGLISH-CHINESE ENCYCLOPEDIA OF PRACTICAL TRADITIONAL CHINESE MEDICINE

Chief Editor	Xu Xiangcai	
Assistants	You Ke	Kang Kai
	Bao Xuequan	Lu Yubin

英汉实用中医药大全

主　编	徐象才	
主编助理	尤可	康凯
	鲍学全	路玉滨

Higher Education Press
高等教育出版社

17 眼科学

	中文	英文	
主 编	蔡华松	陆胜年	
副主编	伊成运	林晓琦	
编 者	王静波	蒋基昌	梁立新
审 校		张志祥	雷希濂

OPHTHALMOLOGY

	English	Chinese
Chief Editor	Lu Shengnian	Cai Huasong
Deputy Chief Editor	Lin Xiaoqi	Yi Chengyun
Editors	Jiang Jichang	Wang Jingbo
	Liang Lixin	
Revisers	Zhang Zhixiang	
	Lei Xilian	

(京)112号

The English-Chinese
Encyclopedia of Practical TCM
Chief Editor   Xu Xiangcai

17
OPHTHALMOLOGY
English Chief Editor   Lu Shengnian
Chinese Chief Editor   Cai Huasong

英汉实用中医药大全
主编   徐象才

17
眼　科　学

中文　　　英文
主编   蔡华松   陆胜年

*

高等教育出版社出版
新华书店总店科技发行所发行
国防工业出版社印刷厂印刷

*

开本 850×1168 1/32 印张 13.125 字数 340 000
1994年8月 第1版 1994年8月 第1次印刷
印数 0 001—3 170
ISBN 7-04-004565-6/R·25
定价 ▇▇▇ 元

The Leading Commission of Compilation and Translation
编译领导委员会

Honorary Director   Hu Ximing
名誉主任委员   胡熙明

Honorary Deputy Directors   Zhang Qiwen   Wang Lei
名誉副主任委员   张奇文   王镭

Director   Zou Jilong
主任委员   邹积隆

Deputy Director   Wei Jiwu
副主任委员   隗继武

Members   Wan Deguang   Wang Yongyan   Wang Maoze
委员   万德光   王永炎   王懋泽
(以姓氏笔划为序)   Wei Guikang   Cong Chunyu   Liu Zhongben
   韦贵康   丛春雨   刘中本
   Sun Guojie   Yan Shiyun   Qiu Dewen
   孙国杰   严世芸   邱德文
   Shang Chichang   Xiang Ping   Zhao Yisen
   尚炽昌   项平   赵以森
   Gao Jinliang   Cheng Yichun   Ge Linyi
   高金亮   程益春   葛琳仪
   Cai Jianqian   Zhai Weimin
   蔡剑前   翟维敏

Advisers   Dong Jianhua   Huang Xiaokai   Geng Jianting
顾问   董建华   黄孝楷   耿鉴庭
   Zhou Fengwu   Zhou Ciqing   Chen Keji
   周凤梧   周次清   陈可冀

The Commission of Compilation and Translation
编译委员会

Director   Xu Xiangcai
主任委员   徐象才

Deputy Directors / 副主任委员

Zhang Zhigang 张志刚	Zhang Wengao 张文高	Jiang Zhaojun 姜兆俊
Qi Xiuheng 秀恒	Xuan Jiasheng 宣家声	Sun Xiangxie 孙祥燮

Members / 委员
(以姓氏笔划为序)

Yu Wenping 于文平	Wang Zhengzhong 王正忠	Wang Chenying 王陈应
Wang Guocai 王国才	Fang Tingyu 方廷钰	Fang Xuwu 方续武
Tian Jingzhen 田景振	Bi Yongsheng 毕永升	Liu Yutan 刘玉檀
Liu Chengcai 刘承才	Liu Jiaqi 刘家起	Liu Xiaojuan 刘晓娟
Zhu Zhongbao 朱忠宝	Zhu Zhenduo 朱振铎	Xun Jianying 寻建英
Li Lei 李磊	Li Zhulan 李竹兰	Xin Shoupu 辛宁璞
Shao Nianfang 邵念方	Chen Shaomin 陈绍民	Zou Jilong 邹积隆
Lu Shengnian 陆胜年	Zhou Xing 周行	Zhou Ciqing 周次清
Zhang Sufang 张素芳	Yang Chongfeng 杨崇峰	Zhao Chunxiu 赵纯修
Yu Changzheng 俞昌正	Hu Zunda 胡遵达	Xu Heying 须鹤瑛
Yuan Jiurong 袁久荣	Huang Naijian 黄乃健	Huang Kuiming 黄奎铭
Huang Jialing 黄嘉陵	Cao Yixun 曹贻训	Lei Xilian 雷希濂
Cai Huasong 蔡华松	Cai Jianqian 蔡剑前	

Preface

I am delighted to learn that THE ENGLISH—CHINESE ENCYCLOPEDIA OF PRACTICAL TRADITIONAL CHINESE MEDICINE will soon come into the world.

TCM has experienced many vicissitudes of times but has remained evergreen. It has made great contributions not only to the power and prosperity of our Chinese nation but to the enrichment and improvement of world medicine. Unfortunately, differences in nations, states and languages have slowed down its spreading and flowing outside China. At present, however, an upsurge in learning, researching and applying Traditional Chinese Medicine (TCM) is unfolding. In order to maximize the effect of this upsurge and to lead TCM, one of the brilliant cultural heritages of the Chinese nation, to the world for it to expand and bring benefit to the people of all nations, Mr. Xu Xiangcai called intellectuals of noble aspirations and high intelligence together from Shandong and many other provinces in China and took charge of the work of both compilation and translation of THE ENGLISH—CHINESE ENCYCLOPEDIA OF PRACTICAL TRADITIONAL CHINESE MEDICINE. With great pleasure, the medical staff both at home and abroad will hail the appearance of this encyclopedia.

I believe that the day when the world's medicine is fully

developed will be the day when TCM has spread throughout the world.

I am pleased to give it my preface.

Prof. Dr. Hu Ximing
    Deputy Ministerof the Ministry of Public Health of the People's Republic of China,
    Director General of the State Administrative Bureau of Traditional Chinese Medicine and Pharmacology,
    President of the World Federation of Acupuncture—Moxibustion Societies,
    Member of China Association of Science & Technology,
    Deputy President of All—China Association of Traditional Chinese Medicine,
    President of China Acupuncture & Moxibustion Society.

December, 1989

Preface

The Chinese nation has been through a long, arduous course of struggling against diseases and has developed its own traditional medicine—Traditional Chinese Medicine and Pharmacology (TCMP). TCMP has a unique, comprehensive, scientific system including both theories and clinical practice. Some thousand years since ito—beginnings, not only has it been well preserved but also continuously developed. It has special advantages, such as remarkable curative effects and few side effects. Hence it is an effective means by which people prevent and treat diseases and keep themselves strong and healthy.

All achievements attained by any nation in the development of medicine are the public wealth of all mankind. They should not be confined within a single country. What is more, the need to set them free to flow throughout the world as quickly and precisely as possible is greater than that of any other kind of science. During my more than thirty years of being engaged in Traditional Chinese Medicine(TCM), I have been looking forward to the day when TCMP will have spread all over the world and made its contributions to the elimination of diseases of all mankind. However it is to be deeply regretted that the pace of TCMP in extending outside China has been unsatisfactory due to the major difficulties in expressing its concepts in foreign languages.

Mr. Xu Xiangcai, a teacher of Shandong College of TCM, has sponsored and taken charge of the work of compilation and translation of The English-Chinese Encyclopedia of Practical Traditional Chinese Medicine—an extensive series. This work is a great project, a large-scale scientific research, a courageous effort and a novel creation. I deeply esteem Mr. Xu Xiangcai and his compilers and translators, who have been working day and night for such a long time, for their hard labor and for their firm and indomitable will displayed in overcoming one difficulty after another, and for their great success achieved in this way. As a leader in the circles of TCM, I am duty-bound to do my best to support them.

I believe this encyclopedia will be certain to find its position both in the history of Chinese medicine and in the history of world science and technology.

Mr. Zhang Qiwen

Member of the Standing Committee of
All-China Association of TCM,
Deputy Head of the Health Department
of Shandong Province.

March, 1990

Publisher's Preface

Traditional Chinese Medicine(TCM) is one of China's great cultural heritages. Since the founding of the People's Republic of China in 1949, guided by the farsighted TCM policy of the Chinese Communist Party and the Chinese government, the treasure house of the theories of TCM has been continuously explored and the plentiful literature researched and compiled. As a result, great success has been achieved. Today there has appeared a world-wide upsurge in the studying and researching of TCM. To promote even more vigorous development of this trend in order that TCM may better serve all mankind, efforts are required to further it throughout the world. To bring this about, the language barriers must be overcome as soon as possible in order that TCM can be accurately expressed in foreign languages.

Thus the compilation and translation of a series of English-Chinese books of basic knowledge of TCM has become of great urgency to serve the needs of medical and educational circles both inside and outside China.

In recent years, at the request of the health departments, satisfactory achievements have been made in researching the expression of TCM in English. Based on the investigation into the history and current state of the research work mentioned above, the English-Chinese Encyclopedia of Practical TCM has been published to meet the needs of extending the knowledge of TCM around the world.

The encyclopedia consists of twenty-one volumes, each dealing with a particular branch of TCM. In the process of compilation, the distinguishing features of TCM have been given close attention and great efforts have been made to ensure that the content is scientific, practical, comprehensive and concise. The chief writers of the Chinese manuscripts include professors or associate professors with at least twenty years of practical clinical and / or teaching experience in TCM. The Chinese manuscript of each volume has been checked and approved by a specialist of the relevant branch of TCM. The team of the translators and revisers of the English versions consists of TCM specialists with a good command of English professional medical translators, and teachers of English from TCM colleges or universities. At a symposium to standardize the English versions, scholars from twenty-two colleges or universities, research institutes of TCM or other health institutes probed the question of how to express TCM in English more comprehensively, systematically and accurately, and discussed and deliberated in detail the English versions of some volumes in order to upgrade the English versions of the whole series. The English version of each volume has been re-examined and then given a final checking.

Obviously this encyclopedia will provide extensive reading material of TCM English for senior students in colleges of TCM in China and will also greatly benefit foreigners studying TCM.

The assiduous efforts of compiling and translating this encyclopedia have been supported by the responsible leaders of the State Education Commission of the People's Republic of China, the State Administrative Bureau of TCM and Pharmacy, and the Education Commission and Health Department of Shandong

Province. Under the direction of the Higher Education Department of the State Education Commission, the leading board of compilation and translation of this encyclopedia was set up. The leaders of many colleges of TCM and pharmaceutical factories of TCM have also given assistance.

We hope that this encyclopedia will bring about a good effect on enhancing the teaching of TCM English at the colleges of TCM in China, on cultivating skills in medical circles in exchanging ideas of TCM with patients in English, and on giving an impetus to the study of TCM outside China.

Higher Education Press
March, 1990

Foreword

The English—Chinese Encyclopedia of Practical Traditional Chinese Medicine is an extensive series of twenty—one volumes. Based on the fundamental theories of traditional Chinese medicine(TCM) and with emphasis on the clinical practice of TCM, it is a semi—advanced English—Chinese academic works which is quite comprehensive, systematic, concise, practical and easy to read. It caters mainly to the following readers: senior students of colleges of TCM, young and middle—aged teachers of colleges of TCM, young and middle—aged physicians of hospitals of TCM, personnel of scientific research institutions of TCM, teachers giving correspondence courses in TCM to foreigners, TCM personnel going abroad in the capacity of lecturers or physicians, those trained in Western medicine but wishing to study TCM, and foreigners coming to China to learn TCM or to take refresher courses in TCM.

Because Traditional Chinese Medicine and Pharmacology is unique to our Chinese nation, putting TCM into English has been the crux of the compilation and translation of this encyclopedia. Owing to the fact that no one can be proficient both in the theories of Traditional Chinese Medicine and Pharmacology and the clinical practice of every branch of TCM, as well as in English, to ensure that the English versions express accurately the inherent meanings of TCM, collective translation measures have been taken. That is, teachers of English familiar with TCM, professional medical translators, teachers or physicians of TCM and even teachers of palaeography with a strong command of English were all invited together to co-translate the Chinese manuscripts and, then, to co-deliberate and discuss the English versions. Finally English-speaking foreigners studying TCM or teaching English in China were asked to polish the English versions. In this way, the skills of the above translators and foreigners were merged to ensure the quality of the English versions. However, even using this method, the uncertainty that the English versions will be wholly accepted still remains. As for the Chinese manuscripts, they do reflect the essence, and give a general picture, of traditional Chinese medicine and pharmacology. It is not asserted, though, that they are perfect, I whole-heartedly look forward to any criticisms or opinions from readers in order to make improvements to future editions.

More than 200 people have taken part in the activities of compiling, translating and revising this encyclopedia. They come from twenty-eight institutions in all parts of China. Among these institutions, there are fifteen colleges of TCM:Shandong, Beijing, Shanghai, Tianjin, Nanjing, Zhejiang, Anhui, Henan, Hubei, Guangxi, Guiyang, Gansu, Chengdu, Shanxi and Changchun, and scientific research centers of TCM such as China Academy of TCM and Shandong Scientific Research Institute of TCM.

The Education Commission of Shandong province has included the compilation and translation of this encyclopedia in its scientific research projects and allocated funds accordingly. The Health Department of Shandong Province has also given financial aid together with a number of pharmaceutical factories of TCM. The subsidization from Jinan Pharmaceutical Factory of

TCM provided the impetus for the work of compilation and translation to get under way.

The success of compiling and translating this encyclopedia is not only the fruit of the collective labor of all the compilers, translators and revisers but also the result of the support of the responsible leaders of the relevant leading institutions. As the encyclopedia is going to be published, I express my heartfelt thanks to all the compilers. translators and revisers for their sincere cooperation, and to the specialists, professors, leaders at all levels and pharmaceutical factories of TCM for their warm support.

It is my most profound wish that the publication of this encyclopedia will take its role in cultivating talented persons of TCM having a very good command of TCM English and in extending, rapidly, comprehensive knowledge of TCM to all corners of the globe.

Chief Editor   Xu Xiangcai

Shandong College of TCM

March, 1990

Contents

Notes 1
1 The Eye and Its Relationship with Zang–Fu Organs and Channels 1
   1.1 The relationship between the eye and *Zang–Fu* organs 1
   1.2 The relationship between the eyes and the Channels 6
   1.3 The theory of Five Orbiculi and Its Application 7
2 Etiology and Pathogenesis 11
   2.1 Etiology 11
   2.2 Pathogenesis 17
3 Methods of Differentiation of Symptoms and Signs Commonly Used in Ophthalmology 24
   3.1 Identification of External and Internal Oculopathy 24
   3.2 Differentiation of Common Symptoms and Signs 25
   3.3 Differentiation of Common Signs of the Fundus 27
4 The Essentials of Treatment 30
   4.1 Internal Treatment 30
   4.2 External Treatment 39
   4.3 Common Medicines of Ophthalmology 45
5 Diseases of the Eyelids 59
   5.1 Hordeolum 60
   5.2 Lid Abscess 63
   5.3 Palpebral Erysipelas 66
   5.4 Palpebral Eczema 70

	5.5 Chalazion	73
	5.6 Blepharitis Cilistis	76
	5.7 Ptosis (Blepharoptosis)	80
6	**Diseases of the Lacrimal Apparatus**	85
	6.1 Dysfunction of the Lacrimal Apparatus	85
	6.2 Chronic Dacryocystitis	89
	6.3 Acute Dacryocystitis	91
7	**Diseases of the Conjunctiva**	95
	7.1 Trachoma	95
	7.2 Acute Catarrhal Conjunctivitis	100
	7.3 Acute Epidemic Conjunctivitis	104
	7.4 Chronic Catarrhal Conjunctivitis	107
	7.5 Phlyctenular Conjunctivitis	111
	7.6 Spring Catarrhal Conjunctivitis	113
	7.7 Pterygium	116
8	**Diseases of the Sclera**	121
	8.1 Scleritis	121
9	**Corneal Diseases**	126
	9.1 Serpiginous Corneal Ulcer	126
	9.2 Herpes Simplex Keratitis	130
	9.3 Deep Keratitis	135
	9.4 Fascicular Keratitis	138
	9.5 Keratomalacia	141
10	**Uveal Diseases**	145
	10.1 Acute Exudative Iridocyclitis	145
	10.2 Chronic Uveitis	148
11	**Diseases of the Lens**	152
	11.1 Senile Cataract	152
	11.2 Traumatic Cataract	156

12	**Glaucoma**	160
	12.1 Acute Angle Closure Glaucoma	160
	12.2 Open-angle Glaucoma	165
13	**Diseases of the Optic Fundus**	170
	13.1 Obstruction of the Central Retinal Vessels	170
	13.2 Retinal Periphlebitis	175
	13.3 Central Serous Choroidal Retinopathy	180
	13.4 Pigmentary Degeneration of the Retina	185
	13.5 Optic Neuritis	188
14	**Diseases of Vitreous**	193
	14.1 Vitreous Opacity	193
15	**Orbital Diseases**	198
	15.1 Acute Orbital Inflammation	198
	15.2 Orbital Pseudotumor	201
16	**Disorders of Ocular Muscles**	205
	16.1 Paralytic Strabismus	205
	16.2 Concomitant Strabismus	208
17	**Ocular Trauma**	212
	17.1 Contusion Injuries	212
	17.2 Penetrating Injuries to the Eye	215
Appendix		219
The English-Chinese Encyclopedia of Practical TCM (Booklist)		399

Notes

OPHTHALMOLOGICAL is the seventeenth of the volumes constituting THE ENGLISH-CHINESE ENCYCLOPEDIA OF PRACTICAL TRADITIONAL CHINESE MEDICINE (TCM). It consists of seventeen chapters and a appendix. Chapters 1-4 introduce the basic theories of ophthalmology of TCM (Traditional Chinese Medicine); Chapters 5-17 deal with the treatments of 41 kinds of oculopathy by way of TCM which will bring about best results. Each kind of eye disease is referred to in terms of modern medicine, and expounded in three aspects: etiology and pathogenesis, clinical manifestations, type and treatment. Various methods are to be applied in the course of treatment, including treating the same disease by different methods, treating different disease with the same therapeutic principle, and differentiation of diseases in conbination with differentiation of symptoms. Commonly used prescriptions of Traditional Chinese Ophthalmology (TCO) are recommended in the appendix.

To Prof. Liu Mianmian of Nanjing Traditional Chinese Medical College, we expressed our thanks for his reading the Chinese manuscripts.

The Editors

1 The Eye and Its Relationship with Zang–Fu Organs and Channels

A human body is an organic unit with its tissues and organs interrelated and mutually influenced as far as the physiologic functions or pathological changes are concerned. Being the optical organ, the eyes are an important component of the human body. They have a close relationship with *Zang–Fu* organs, channels, *Qi* and blood. If dysfunction occurs in any of the above four fields, it will be reflected immediately in the eyes, thus leading to eye diseases. On the other hand, eye diseases may influence the related viscera through the channels, *Qi* and blood, leading to dysfunction of the viscera and a general reaction of the whole body might follow.

Therefore when we study the etiology and pathogenesis of eye diseases and try to determine the treatment, we should not merely consider the local signs but have to follow wholism, that is, to make overall observations and comprehensive analyses of the relationship between the eyes and *Zang–Fu* organs, channels and collaterals.

1.1 The relationship between the eye and *Zang–Fu* organs

The ability of the eyes is to see objects and distinguish colors. This function is completely attributed to nutrition by essential *Qi* of the *Zang–Fu* organs. The essential *Qi* of the five solid and six hollow organs flows upwards to support the eye's vision. Dysfunction of the *Zang–Fu* organs will restrict the essential–*Qi* from being transmitted to the eyes, which will affect vision and may cause eye diseases.

The liver has its specific opening in the eyes. The visual ability of one's eyes depends on the blood stored in the liver. The liver–*Qi* flows to the eyes, therefore, the normal function of the liver enables the eyes to distinguish various colors. The liver is in charge of storing blood. Its capability to store blood enables it to regulate the circulating blood volume. The liver also possesses the function of dispersing and regulating the flow of *Qi* in the body.

When the liver is full of blood, the liver–*Qi* flows freely, and the refined nutritive essence in the liver activated by *Qi* is transferred to the eyes. This continual supply of nutrient maintains normal function of vision.

If liver–blood is too insufficient and liver–*Yin* or Liver–*Qi* are too deficient, they fail to transport enough refined essence to the eyes, and poor or blurred vision due to lack of nourishment may occur. Stagnation of liver–*Qi* may cause disorder in the *Qi* system. Dysfunction of the liver in dispersing leads to adverse upward movement of liver–*Qi* which in turn causes the blood to follow the *Qi* up, attacking the upper part of the body, resulting in stagnancy of *Qi* and blood, or extravasation of the blood. Either of the two cases may cause eye diseases.

The liver and the gallbladder are interior–exteriorly related. The liver–*Qi* overflows to the gallbladder and accumulates there to form what is called bile. The bile infiltrates and ascends to the eyes where it accumulats to form vitreous and aqueous humor which nourishes the pupil and gives good vision. When the heat of the gallbladder is excessive, it will burn the vitreous and aqueous humor to make them turbid. This will impair nourishment of the pupil and cause blurred vision.

All blood flows from and to the heart, All channels are connected with the eyes. The heart governs the blood and blood vessels of the body. Activated by the heart—Qi, blood in the vessels circulates through the whole body. When the blood flows to the eyes, it provides them with nourishment to maintain normal visual function. That is to say, eyes can see only when nurtured by blood.

If the heart—fire burns vigorously and impairs the vessels, extravasation of stagnation of blood will happen, resulting in discontinuance of blood supply. Hypopsia or even ablepsia may then occur due to lack of nourishment of the eye. When heart—Qi is sufficient and its function is normal, one is full of vigour, which will result in bright and agile eyes. Insufficiency of heart—Qi or blood will bring about dysfunction of the heart in governing blood circulation, leading to failure of enough blood to flow to the eyes. As a result, blurred vision will occur with weary and lusterless eyes. So the eyes are the messenger and external orifice of the heart.

The heart and the small intestine are interior—exteriorly related. The function of the latter is to separate the refined substances from the dross. The refined substance, including body fluid and essential substances from food—staff, is absorbed by the small intestine and carried to the spleen. Then the spleen distributes these substances to the eyes, so that the eyes look moist and lustrous, agile and clear in vision. With dysfunction of the small intestine in separating the refined substance from the dross, poor nourishment may cause dryness and discomfort of the eyes. Hence blurred vision may occur.

The kidney controls water metabolism, receives and stores the essence of all the *Zang* and *Fu* organs. Visual function depends mainly on the nourishment from the essence of the *Zang* and *Fu* organs, and the kidney is the very place where essence is stored. Therefore there is a close relationship between the abundance of essence stored in the kidney and the normality of visual function. Although the liver has its specific opening in the eyes, the kidney controls the visual function of them. The eyes can function normally only when the kidney—Qi is in normal condition and the kidney essence is sufficiently distributed to the eyes. Deficiency of the kidney and insufficiency of the essence stored in the kidney may bring about blurred vision.

The kidney stores vital essence from which marrow is formed. The brain known as the sea of marrow is connected with the eyes by means of ocular connectors, Hence, insufficiency of the sea of marrow attributable to deficiency of kidney causes blurred vision.

The function of the kidney in controlling water metabolism plays an important role in distribution, retention and excretion of water within the body. In the case of normal metabolism, the water and body fluid are transformed into tears, aqueous humor to moisten and nourish the eyeballs. Dysfunction of water metabolism, however, may cause water retention within the body, which may attack the eye, leading to blurred vision and metamorphopsia.

The kidney and the urinary bladder are interior—exteriorly related. The urinary bladder has the function of storing and discharging urine. When this organ functions normally, the refined-essence flows up to the eye and the turbid *Qi* goes down to be discharged off the body; the eyes being bright. Dysfunction of the urinary bladder may cause failure in separating the refined essence from the dross, resulting in retention of water. Lingering retention of water may produce heat. When this damp-heat attacks the eyes, blurred, poor or muscegenetic vision may occur.

The *Qi* of the five *Zang*-organs flows up to the nine orifices. And *Zang*-organs receive *Qi* from the six *Fu* organs which in turn receive *Qi* from the stomach. Thus all the *Qi* of *Zang* and *Fu* organs actually comes from the spleen and goes up to the eyes. Therefore the eyes have a very close relationship with the spleen and the stomach.

The spleen is in charge of transportation and transformation, sending nutrients upward while the stomach is responsible for sending digested food downward. When the two organs function normally, the essence of lucid-*Yang* flows up to nourish the eyes. Thus clear vision is obtained. As the muscles of the eyes obtain nutrients, the eyeballs will move freely and the eyelids open or close easily. On the contrary, failure in bringing up lucid-*Yang* gives rise to lack of nourishment of the eyes and failure in sending down turbid-*Yin* may affect the eyes. This will bring about various eye diseases. The spleen governs the blood, which nourishes the eyes. Because of this function of the spleen, blood circulates within the vessels of the eyes without extravasation to nourish the eyes. If there appears failure to keep the blood flow within the vessels due to insufficiency of the spleen, hemorrage diseases of the eyes will ensue.

The lung is in charge of dispersion, and distributes *Qi*, blood and body fluid to the eye. The lung also has purifying and descending function, which conducts fluid downward to the urinary bladder. When the dispersing and descending function of the lung is normal, blood circulates freely to warm and nourish the eyes, which protects the eyes from being attacked by pathogens. Dysfunction of the lung may lead to disorder of *Qi*, stagnation of *Qi* and blood bringing about eye diseases.

The lung and the large intestine are interior—exteriorly related and influence each other in functioning. If heat accumulates in the large intestine, obstruction of *Qi* in *Fu* organs may lead to failure of the lung—*Qi* to descending function which may also cause eye diseases. When the purifying and descending function of the lung is impaired, *Fu*—*Qi* pushes forward so feebly as to cause dysfunction of the large intestine in transmission. If this condition lasts long, excessive heat will arise and the resulting excessive heat in *Yang*—*ming* may also cause eye diseases.

1.2 The relationship between the eyes and the Channels

The blood and *Qi* of the 12 channels and the about 365 collaterals are all distributed to the head, the face and the orifices of the body. The essence and energy are distributed to the eyes to form visual function. The channels and the collaterals have the functions of connecting the *Zang* organs with *Fu* organs, correlating the interior with the exterior of the body. They also transmit *Qi* and blood. The transport of the essence of the *Zang* and *Fu* organs to the eyes depends upon the transimitting function of the channels.

The relation between the eyes and the channels can be classified into three forms:

Firstly, the channels have direct connections with the eyes. For example, the Liver Channel of Foot *Jueyin* is connected with the ocular connectors. The Gallbladder Channel of Foot *Shaoyang* starts from the outer canthus while the Urinary Bladder Channel of Foot *Taiyang* from the inner canthus. The Stomach Channel of Foot *Yangming* enters into the inner canthus.

Secondly, the collaterals connect with the eyes. For example, the collaterals of the Heart Channel of Hand *Shaoyin* connect with the ocular connectors. Collaterals of the Small Intestine Channel of Hand *Shaoyang* and *Sanjiao* Channel of Hand *Shaoyang* enter at the outer canthi.

Thirdly, other channels through large collaterals connect with the eyes.

In pathology, affection by six external etiological factors or internal injury caused by persistant and violent emotions can traverse inward from the eyes to impair internal organs through channels or from internal organs to impair the eyes.

1.3 The theory of Five Orbiculi and Its Application

The theory of five orbiculi is based on "Canon of Internal Medicine", which indicates the relationship of the various parts of the eye with *Zang-Fu* organs and lays a solid foundation for the theory of the five orbiculi. According to this theory, the eye can be divided into five parts: flesh orbiculus, blood orbiculus, *Qi* orbiculus, wind orbiculus and water orbiculus, all of which correspond to the five *Zang* organs respectively and in this way it explains the anatomy, physiology and pathology of the eyes and their relationship with *Zang—Fu* organs.

The contents of the five—orbiculi theory are enriched and perfected with the development, replenishment and perfection of the theory of *Zang—Fu*. At present, this theory is still widely used in clinical diagnosis and treatment based on overall analysis of symptoms and signs.

Flesh orbiculus refers to the eyelids including the skin of the eyelids, the subcutaneous tissues, muscles, the outer plate, and the palpebral conjunctiva. It is the outer portion of the eye. Its function is in charge of the opening and closing of the eyes. It corresponds to the spleen which is in charge of the muscles. Therefore it is called flesh orbiculus.

The spleen and the stomach are interior—exteriorly related. When the functions of the spleen and the stomach are in normal condition, the color of the eyelids is also normal, and the eyelids can open and close freely. If hypofunction of the spleen results in insufficiency of *Qi* in middle—*Jiao,* the eyelids are lax and difficult to lift due to poor nourishment. Redness and erosion on the margin of the eyelids usually attribute to the retention of pathogenic damp—heat in the spleen and the stomach. Redness, swelling and pain of the eyelids are caused by excessive—stomach fire and heat—accumulation in *Yangming—Fu* organs.

Blood orbiculus refers to inner and outer canthi and the skin thereabout, the semilunar fold, lacrimal caruncle, lacrimal duct, dacryocyst and part of the conjunctiva and sclera near the canthi. The canthi correspond to the heart. They are called blood orbiculi because the heart governs blood circulation. When the heart functions normally, blood governed by the heart circulates freely and the skin of the canthi is moist and sheen. But when the heart—fire flames up to the eyes, redness and soreness of the puncta lacrimals may occur.

Qi orbiculus refers to the white of the eye, i.e. the bulbar conjunctiva, and sclera, *Qi* orbiculus corresponds to the lung which governs *Qi*. Therefore it is termed *Qi* orbiculus. The texture of the sclera is tough. It protects the eye tissues. Sufficiency of lung—*Qi* protects the body against disease. The bulbar conjunctiva is white and moist when lung—*Yin* is abundant, otherwise it becomes dry and looks gloomy.

Wind orbiculus refers to the black of the eye, i.e. the cornea, which is tough and transparent. The cornea connecting with the sclera forms the superficial layer of the eyeball. It corresponds to the liver which is in charge of wind. Therefore it is called wind orbiculus. When liver—*Qi* is regular and liver—*Yin* is sufficient, the black of the eye is clear with its surface smooth and the eyes can obtain good vision. But when there exists pathogenic heat in the liver channel and it attacks the eyes, nephelium, pancorneal opacity and blurred vision may occur.

Water orbiculus refers to the pupil including aqueous humor, iris, pupil, lens, vitreous body, retina, optic nerves and choroid. The pupil corresponds to the kidney which is in charge of water metabolism. Therefore it is called water orbiculus and it is one of the most important parts of vision. When the kidney is full of essence and the eyes are well nourished, the pupil is clear and it contracts or expands freely to ensure clear vision. Insufficiency of kidney essence and consumption of body fluid result in dim pupil and the pupils may even gradually turn whitish.

In short, the theory of the five orbiculi has clearly defined the relationship between the eyes and the whole body and also the corresponding relationship of the orbiculi with the *Zang—Fu* organs. Therefore, we can also diagnose the pathogenic changes of the *Zang—Fu* organs by examining the symptoms shown in various parts of the eye.

2 Etiology and Pathogenesis

2.1 Etiology

Etiology refers to the causative factors of diseases. The eyes, which contact directly with the external environment and at the same time are closely linked with *Zang-Fu* organs and channels, are liable to become diseased due to affection by pathogenic factors inside and outside the body. The etiology of Traditional Chinese Ophthalmology attaches much importance to the interior-exterior pathogenic factors and it also lays much emphasis on vital-*Qi*, that is, the body's resistance factors. A person is inflicted with pathogenic factors when his body resistance is debilitated. The occurrence and recovery of eye diseases are reflections of the struggle between the vital-*Qi* and pathogenic factors.

Eye diseases can be caused by exogenous, endogenous or non-endo-exopathogenic factors. Exogenous pathogenic factors are wind, cold, summer heat, dampness, dryness and fire, and in addition, epidemics may also be included. Of the six pathogenic factors, wind and fire attack the eyes most commonly. Endogenous pathogenic factors refer to joy, anger melancholy, anxiety, grief, fear and terror. These are the seven modes of emotion. Internal impairment by seven emotions due to emotional stress or upsets may cause disturbance in the functions of *Zang-Fu* organs and derangement of *Qi* and blood, resulting in eye diseases. Non-endo-exopathogenic factors include trauma, improper diet, overwork, etc.

Six Pathogenic Factors

Under normal conditions, wind, cold, summer-heat, dampness, dryness, fire are called "six types of *Qi* ". They are known as "six exopathogenic factors " when they are excessive, insufficient or in disharmony with the season.

All the six pathogenic factors may invade the body from the exterior via the skin, mouth or nose to the interior or along the channels attacking the upper part of the body and causing eye diseases. Or they may attack the eye directly, resulting in disease. The six pathogenic factors may assault the body singly or in collabortion. They are closely related to seasonal changes and usually cause external eye diseases.

Wind: Wind is a *Yang* pathogenic factor, characterized by upward and out-ward dispersion. The ancients said: " It is the upper part of the body that is easily affected by pathogenic wind" . The eyes are apt to be affected by an attack of pathogenic wind because they are on the superficial and at the upper part of the body. Eye diseases caused by wind usually affect the eyelid, canthus, the bulbar conjunctiva the cornea and iris.

In the six pathogenic factors, wind is the leading causative factor of many diseases not only causing eye diseases singly but also acting as a precursor for invasion of the other five pathogenic factors: it may attack the eyes in company of cold, dampness, dryness and fire, leading to eye diseases.

Wind is speedy and apt to change. Therefore, eye diseases caused by wind are marked by sudden onset and rapid changes. For example, eye diseases, such as psreudo membranous conjuctivitis, nebula, redness, swelling and soreness due to invasion of pathogenic wind, all have sudden onset. The eye diseases caused by pathogenic wind may manifest themselves as: itching, discomfort, photophobia, lacrimation, conjunctival congestion, nebula, edema of the eyelids, ptosis of upper eyelid, paralytic strabismus, etc.

Fire: Fire is *Yang* in nature characterized by flaring up. Therefore it is apt to attack the eyes and cause eye diseases. Other pathogenic factors attacking the body are apt to turn into fire. Fire is the motive force of life. When fire is in its normal condition, it is vital−*Qi,* whereas when it is in its abnormal condition, it is pathogenic heat. Heat is the initial form of fire while fire is the extreme form of heat. Hence it is difficult to separate fire from heat. Fire is *Yang* in nature while *Yang* is characterized by rising. Fire and heat, sharing the same nature, all tend to flare up to attack the head and eyes, thus causing diseases.

The diseases caused by pathogenic fire or heat manifest themselves as redness, swollon eyelids and ulceration, aversion to heat, photophobia, discomfort and pain, inability to open eyelids, conjunctival congestion, burning and urticant sensation, epiphora with hot sensation, abundance of sticky, yellowish eye secretion, redness, swelling and pain of the eyelids, tenderness, chemosis and hyperemia and ecchymosis of bulbar conjunctiva, nebula, ulcer or protuberance of the cornea. These symptoms usually lead to hypopyon, miosis, sudden loss of vision, phyphemia, etc.

Dampness: It is a *Yin* pathogen characterized by heaviness and turbidity, viscosity and stagnation. *Yang−Qi* is easily affected by dampness leading to disturbance in ascending and dispersing upward. Therefore the onset of the disease due to affection of dampness is usually slow and the disease is chronic and intractable with remissions and exacerbations.

Determined by the abundance or scarity of *Yang−Qi* reserved in the patient, dampness which has invaded into the body may bring about heat or cold, leading to dampness−heat retention or stagnation of cold−dampness. Diseases caused by dampness manifest themselves as tears with mucopurulent secretion, marginal blepharitis, wet itching and small vesicles, yellowish fluid flowing out after diabrosis, scarring, xanthosis or hyperemia of the bulbar conjunctiva, blurred vision, retinal edema or subretinal exudation.

Cold: Cold is *Yin* in nature and characterized by stagnation. The invasion of external cold pathogens is apt to damage *Yang−Qi*. If *Yang−Qi* is deficient, the eyes will lack warmth and nourishment, resulting in cold−epiphora and blurred vision. Pathogenic cold stagnates within the skin, muscles and blood vessels of the eyelids, causing stagnation of *Qi* and blood. This may manifest as purple swelling eyelids, the vessels of the bulbar conjunctiva are purple or pink in color. As pathogenic cold invades and damages vessels and channels, the patient will feel uncomfortable of the lids. with a tense sensation.

Dryness: Dryness is *Yang* in nature and characterized by dryness astringency and is apt to consume the body fluids. Diseases caused by pathogenic dryness manifest themselves as dryness and discomfort of the eyes, frequent nictation, caked eye secretion, hyperemia of bulbar conjunctiva, dull eyes or even with folds at the eye surface, As time passes, pancorneal opacity may occur, leading to blurred vision.

Summer heat: It is *Yang* in nature and characterized by extreme heat and is apt to consume body fluids. Usually summer heat is accompanied by dampness, causing diseases manifested as conjunctival congestion, swelling, soreness, blurred vision, palpebral eczema vesicle, erosion ulcer, etc.

The endogenous wind, fire, cold, dampness and dryness develop from dysfunction and disturbance of the *Zang-Fu* organs, blood, *Qi* and body fluids. Their manifestations will be stated in the next chapter.

Diseases caused by only one of the six pathogenic factors are less frequently seen. In general, many pathogenic factors collaborate in causing diseases, of which wind-heat and wind-fire attack most commonly.

As the human body is an organic whole, the eyes have a close relationship with the whole body. Hence, disease of the eye caused by any or some of the six pathogenic factors is not only indicated by a local signs of the eye but often complicated by certain general symptoms of the body. Likewise, a general disease of the body caused by the six pathogenic factors often presents certain symptoms of the eye or complicated by some eye diseases. Thus in clinical differentiation of syndromes in ophthalmology, we must analyse both general and local signs and symptoms.

Epidemics

They are extremely infectious pathogenic factors. The epidemics which cause eye diseases are of warmth and heat in nature. The characteristics of the disease caused by epidemics are sudden onset, rage, rapid changes, intense infectivity and pandemic tendency. The clinical manifestations are chemosis and hyperemia of bulbar conjunctiva, palpebral edema, frequent epiphora with hot sensation, photophobia and aversion to heat, and nebula, ophthalmalgia in severe casess.

Seven Emotions

Normally, emotional changes are the manifestations of mental activities, while the material basis of them is the essence of *Zang-Fu*. Violent emotional changes may influence the normal functions of *Zang-Fu*, causing disturbance of visceral function and abnormal circulation of *Qi*. And the essence may thus fail to nourish the eyes, leading to eye diseases or eye symptoms of general disease of the body.

Emotional stress may lead to disorder of *Qi*, causing stagnated *Qi*, which may be turned into flaring-up fire.

The symptoms in the eye caused by emotional disturbance are various: Frequent epiphora, discomfort and slight congestion, swelling pain of the eyeball, blurred vision, nebula of the cornea, sudden loss of vision, optic atrophy, five-colored glaucoma.

Improper Diet

Food intake provides basic materials for the body to maintain its vital activities. Irregular and improper diet may impair the function of the spleen and stomach. The spleen and stomach provide the material basis for the acquired constitution. The essence of *Zang-Fu* organs is received from the spleen and stomach and flows up to the eyes. Insufficient food intake will fail to provide the necessary material for the manufacture of *Qi* and blood. In the long run, exhaustion of vital essence of *Zang-Fu* may occur. Superfluous diet will inevitably impair the spleen and stomach, leading to failure in manufacture of blood and vital essence due to dysfunction of transportation and transformation. As a result, eye disease may occur since deficient vital essence fails to nourish the eyes. The clinical manifestations include ptosis of the upper eyelid, blurred vision, optic atrophy, etc. Eating too much of fatty, pungent, hot-roasted or deep-fried foods, not to mention overdrinking, may cause retention of dampness-heat or phlegm in the spleen and stomach. They attack the eyes with such signs and symptoms as palpebral swelling pain, marginal blepharitis, subcutaneous nodules. ulcers, etc. Eye diseases due to attacks by dampness manifest themselves as blurred vision, retinal edema, subretinal exudation, preretinal hemorrhage. Children's prolonged overindulgence in a particular kind of food may lead to deficiency of *Qi* and blood, which fails to nourish the eyes resulting in nyctalopia, or eye disorders due to malnutrition.

Overstrain

Overstrain mainly refers to extravagant use of physical strength, mental power and vision and intemperate sexual intercourses to such an extent that it causes deficiency of blood and exhaustion of *Yin* essence. This lack of nourishment may lead to deficiency of essence and flaring up of fire of deficiency type, resulting in eye diseases ,such as optic atrophy, blurred vision, cataract, etc.

2.2 Pathogenesis

Pathogenesis refers to the mechanism for the occurrence, development and change of a disease. In discussing pathogenesis of eye diseases, we must not leave out the concept that the body is an organic whole. Eye diseases may occur when pathogenic factors cause imbalance of *Yin* and *Yang*, disturbance in circulation of *Qi* and dysfunctions of *Zang-Fu* organs, channels, *Qi* and blood. The individual constitutions are different from each other, therefore the etiology of the disease varies and the pahogenesis becomes very complicated.

Dysfunction of *Zang–Fu* organs

Dysfunction of the liver and gallbladder: Clinically, most eye diseases due to dysfunction of the liver and gallbladder fall into excess syndrome and are mostly caused by upward attacks of pathogenic fire or steaming dampness–heat. If they happen to be deficiency syndrome, they are in most cases due to deficiency of liver–*Yin* or of liver blood. Hyperactivity of fire due to *Yin* deficiency or upstirring of liver wind is usually seen in mixed syndromes of deficiency and excess. When there is fire in the liver and gallbladder, fire syndrome caused by stagnation of liver–*Qi*, and transmission of pathogenic factors to *Shao–Yang* and *Jue–Yin* channels, the upward adverse flow of *Qi* and fire may attack the head and the eyes, resulting in impairment of wind–orbiculus. The manifestations are conjunctival congestion, swelling pain, photophobia and epiphora with hot sensation, nebula, ulcer of the cornea and miosis.

When heat invades the blood and burns the vessels in the eyes, extravasation of blood and hemorrhage may occur in the eyes. Stagnation of liver–*Qi* causes dysfunction of the dispersing and discharging role of the liver, resulting in stagnation of vital–*Qi* and disturbance of blood and body fluid circulation. The manifestations are conjunctival congestion and blurred vision, a hard eyeball with distending pain which may involve the forehead and hypopsia. Lack of nutrition to the tendons and vessels due to stagnation of *Qi* and blood leads to oculogyration pain, blurred vision and sudden loss of vision. When there is dampness–heat in the liver and gallbladder, the steaming dampness due to retention of dampness–heat may attack the eyes, or turbid *Qi* can flow up to clog the head and the eyes, affecting the normality of the head and the eye with hyperemia of the bulbar conjunctiva and purulent keratitis. The eyes may lack of nourishment due to insufficiency of liver blood, bringing about dryness and discomfort of the eyes, blurred vision or even blindness.

Insufficiency of liver blood in children may lead to nyctalopia and dryness of the eyes without lustre. Hyperactivity of the liver—*Yang* due to deficiency of the liver—*Yin* may cause sore eyes or hyperemia of the conjunctiva with blurred vision. Deficiency of the liver—*Yin* leads to flaring up of fire of deficiency type. And endogenous wind of the liver stirs up. The fire and wind stand together and attack the eyes, resulting in headache, distention in the eyes, strabismus and fickering eyelids.

Dysfunction of the kidney and urinary bladder: Eye diseases caused by dysfunction of kidney and urinary bladder mostly fall into deficiency syndrome: Deficiency of kidney—*Yin* or of kidney—*Yang* .Only a few are of excess syndrome. Because the liver and kidney have a common source, deficiency of liver—*Yin* and kidney—*Yin* result in poor nourishment of *Yin*—essence to the head and eyes, causing opacity in the eyes, vague pain in the eyeball, strained pain when the eyes are rolling, hypopsia and dizziness. Insufficiency of kidney—*Yang* leads to hypofunction of the organs' role in warming and transformation. Thus the eyes, lacking warmth and nourishment, are dim. Deficiency of vital fire due to *Yang* insufficiency causes failure in warming and dispersing water, resulting in retention of water. The retarted water overflows within the skin and muscles of the eyelid, leading to palpebral edema while overflowing of water in the eyes may lead to retinal edema, subretinal exudation or even retinal detachment. Disturbance of *Qi* transformation due to accumulation of heat in the urinary bladder results in attack by steaming dampness—heat, thus causing conjunctival congestion, headache, and gloomy look of the white part of the eye.

Dysfunction of the heart and small intestine: In eye diseases caused by dysfunction of the heart and small intestine, excess syndromes are mostly induced by the hyperactivity of the heart fire while deficiency syndromes mostly suggest deficiency of heart *Yin*. Flaring heart fire attacks the eyes and burns blood vessels, resulting in invasion to the blood system by heat. This results in prickling—like pain in the eyeball, hyperemia of bulbar conjunctiva in the region of inner canthi, distended blood vessels, thickening pterygium, and in drastic cases extravasation of blood marked by subconjunctival ecchymosis, hemalopia and hypopsia. Excessive pathogenic fire in the body may also cause ulcer of the eyes with pus. Poor nourishment of the eyes due to deficiency of *Yin*—fluid and blood may cause sensation of dryness and itching and blurred vision. Flaring—up fire of deficiency type may bring about slight congestion of the conjunctiva, photophobia and lacrimation.

Dysfunction of the spleen and stomach: The pathogenesis of eye diseases caused by dysfunction of the spleen and stomach is mostly related to excessiveness of stomach fire, dampness—heat in the spleen and stomach and insufficiency of the spleen and *Qi*, and failure of the spleen to keep the blood flowing within the vessels. As the stomach fire is exessive, it will move upward along the channels to attack eyes, resulting in local stagnation of *Qi* and blood and blockage of the vessels and causing such symptoms as hyperemia of the bulbar conjunctiva, edema, hard swelling eyelid, or even abscess of the eyelid. Excessive heat in *Yang—ming* results in pathogenic heat attacking the eyes, burning the iris, leading to turbid aqueous humor and miosis.

If dampness—heat accumulates in the spleen and stomach, the excessive heat may steam the dampness forming turbid *Qi* which flows to the upper part of the body, blocking the seven orifices, and causing retinal edema, subretinal exudation, preretinal hemorrhage and blurred vision. Dampness—heat accumulated in the eyelid results in stagnation of *Qi* and blood which may bring about papilledema, folliculosis, small blisters on the margin, blepharitis marginalis and scarring, or even redness and swelling pain of the eyelid, and ulceration with pus. Accumulation of phlegm—dampness in the spleen results in insufficiency of spleen—*Yang*, impairment of water metabolism, leading to dampness—heat accumulation in the body, blocking the vessels and channels of the eyelid. This may cause swelling of the eyelid with bearing down sensation and, in protracted cases, a mass will form.

Hypofunction of the spleen leads to insufficiency of blood transformation, resulting in poor nourishment of the tendons, vessels, muscles of the eyelid. This may cause blepharochalasis, or blepharptosis. Failure of the spleen to keep the blood flowing within the vessels results in extravasation in the eyes, which causes blurred, muscaegenetic vision in mild cases, and lose of vision in severe cases.

Dysfunction of the lung and large intestine: In eye diseases caused by dysfunction of the lung and large intestine, the excess syndrome is usually attributed to attacks on the lungs by external pathogenic factors which result in disturbance of dispersing and descending functions of the lung. While the deficiency syndrome is usually due to insufficiency of the lung—*Yin*.

Attack to the lung by wind heat disturbs the lung's dispersing and descending function, and impairs its function in distribution. This may cause obstruction of blood and *Qi* in the vessels of the eyes, resulting in bulbar conjunctival congestion, tortuosity and distention of the vessels. Water retention in the eyes due to failure of transporting water to the urinary bladder causes distending pain in the eyes and bulbar conjunctiva edema. Excessive heat of the lung attacks the eyes, causing aversion of the eyes to heat, photophobia, profuse viscose secretions, bulbar conjunctiva congestion and edema, or even hyperemia of sclera with dark blue color. Invasion to the blood system by heat causes abnormal flow of blood and impairs the vessels and channels, leading to bulbar conjunctival hemorrhage. Flaring—up of asthenic fire due to insufficiency of lung—*Yin* may cause sensation of dryness, discomfort, dull pain of the eyes, caked eye secretions and prolonged bulbar conjunctival congestion.

Dysfunction of *Qi* and blood

Deficiency of *Qi* and *Qi* collapse: Failure of *Yang Qi* to rise and distribute due to deficiency of vital—*Qi* causes poor nourishment of the eyes, incapability of the body resistance to protect the body against disease, dysfunction of the organs' role in governing and warming. These may mainly manifest in the eye as blepharoptosis, epiphora with cold sensation, prolonged corneal ulcer, visual fatigue, etc.

Stagnation of *Qi* and reversed flow of *Qi*: Impeded circulation of *Qi*, abnormal ascension and descension of *Qi* may lead to eye diseases. Obstruction of the vessels and channels due to dysfunction of lung—*Qi* may cause bulbar conjunctival congestion and nodular projections. When the liver—Qi is stagnated and depressed, the hyperactive liver—Qi may attack the upper part of the body or cause fire syndrome. During the upward adverse movement of Qi and fire ,the blood may attack upward with them as well. When the fire burns the vessels the blood may extravasate from the vessels, resulting in distent pain in the eyeball, blurred vision, optical fundus hemorrhage and dull pain when the eyes are rolling.

Blood heat: Heat in the blood speeds up blood circulation which is likely to cause red eyelid, swelling pain with hot sensation in the eyes. When pathogenic heat in blood impairs the vessels, resulting in extravasation, the consequent symptoms in the eye may be bulbar conjunctiva hemorrhage, optical fundus hemorrhage.

Blood stasis: Stagnation of blood in the eyes may lead to blepharal cyanosis, bulbar conjunctiva and sclera congestion presenting a dark blue color. Obstruction of the vessels of retina leads to retinal edema, hemorrhage, blurred vision and continuous severe pain at definite spot.

Deficiency of blood: Deficiency of blood results in failure of blood to nourish the head and eyes marked by dizziness, poor vision, pale eyelid, sensation of dryness and discomfort, inability to use one's vision continuously, dry and lustreless eyes, dull pain in the eyeball and itching from time to time.

3 Methods of Differentiation of Symptoms and Signs Commonly Used in Ophthalmology

The methods of differentiation of symptoms and signs commonly used in ophthalmology are similar to those of internal medicine. But there are still some peculiarities in this branch. Generally, differentiation of local symptoms and signs are mainly used in acute eye diseases while differentiation of general symptoms and signs are mainly used in chronic eye diseases. Here are several methods commonly used for differentiation of local symptoms and signs.

3.1 Identification of External and Internal Oculopathy

External Oculopathy: This refers to the diseases on the surface of eyeball or its accessory organs. External oculopathy is usually caused by invasion of any of the six external phathogenic factors or by internal accumulation of phlegm—damp, insufficiency of the spleen—Qi, deficiency of the liver and the kidney, trauma or other factors. The characteristics of external oculopathy are acute onset, and quick development, marked external symptoms and signs such as red and swelling eyelids, hyperemia of the bulbar conjunctiva, opacitas cornea, photophobia, lacrimation, etc. Generally speaking, acute external oculopathies are grouped as excess syndrome while the chronic ones mainly as deficiency syndrome.

Internal Oculopathy: This refers to the diseases which involve the tissues and the visual nerves inside the eyeball. Internal oculopathy is caused by persistent and violent emotions, overstrain, trauma, etc resulting in dysfunction of viscera, channels, *Qi* and blood. Internal oculopathy manifests itself mainly in visual dysfunction, usually with no external signs. Internal oculopathy usually falls into deficiency syndrome though it may also belong in mixed syndrome of deficiency and excess.

3.2 Differentiation of Common Symptoms and Signs

Observation of the vision: Blurred vision with ciliary congestion or mixed congestion is mainly caused by exposure to pathogenic wind—heat or excessive fire of the liver and gallbladder. Despite of absence of external symptoms and signs gradual drop of vision, muscaegenetic vision and metamorphosia, usually suggest stagnation of phlegm—dampness, deficiency of the liver and kidney or deficiency of blood and *Qi*. Though the eye is normal externally, sudden drop of vision is usually a sign of stagnation of blood and *Qi*, bleeding due to blood—heat, excessive fire of the liver and the gallbladder or hyperactivity of fire due to *Yin*—deficiency.

Observation of redness and swelling: Palpebral redness, swelling and pain are mainly due to retention of pathogenic heat in the spleen and the stomach. Palpebral swelling without redness or pain is due to *Yang* deficiency of the spleen and the kidney, resulting in water and dampness attacking upwards. Redness, swelling and erosion of the eyelid are due to dampness—heat retention in the body. Livid eyelid is due to blood stasis.

Hyperemia of the bulbar conjunctiva, lacrimation, profuse secretion are usually caused by the attack of exogenous wind—heat or heat of excess type of the lung channel. Edema of bulbar conjunctiva without hyperemia is due to dysfunction of the lung—*Qi*. Ciliary congestion or mixed congestion is due to heat of excess type in the liver—gallbladder. Localized congestion is caused by heat retention in the lung channel and obstruction of the lung—*Qi*.

Observation of pain and itching: Usually, sudden pain indicates excess syndrome while persistent pain indicates deficiency syndrome. Pain but the patient denial of perssing and with a desire for cold is caused by heat of excess type. Pain relieved by pressing and intolerance of cold is due to cold of deficiency type. Day—time pain is *Yang*, while night—time pain is *Yin*. Severe of distending pain is due to hyperactivity of fire of the liver and gallbladder. Dull pain is due to hyperactivity of fire caused by deficiency of *Yin*.

Itching of the eyes usually suggests wind and it can be classified into deficiency type and excess type. Itching of the eyes may also by caused by allergy to food or medicines. Unbearable itching with lacrimation, hyperemia of the bulbar conjunctiva are due to the affection of exogenous wind—heat. Itching with red, swelling eyelid and erosion of the skin is due to dampness—heat in the spleen and stomach complicated with invasion of pathogenic wind. When the disease is about to recover, itching is caused by free circulation of the blood and *Qi*. Slight intermittent itching is caused by endopathic wind due to deficiency of blood.

Observation of the eye secretion and tears: Profuse viscid,

yellowish discharge is due to hyperactivity of the noxious heat. Copious indurated eye secretion is due to the heat of excess type of the lung channel. Watery unindurated eye secretion is due to heat of deficiency type of the lung channel. Sticky eye secretion is due to accumulation of dampness—heat. Tears are classified into two types: cold and warm. A large amount of warm tears is due to pathogenic wind—heat or trauma. Epiphora induced by wind or cold epiphora is due to deficiency of the liver and kidney.

Observation of the nebula and membrane: Nebulal refers to diseases of the cornea. New nebula is charaterized by inflammatory opacity. If it is stellate or arborescent it is caused by wind—heat on the liver channel. If an ulcer is formed or complicated with iritis, it is due to excessiveness of the noxious heat. Stubborn ulcer is due to residence of pathogenic factors as a result of debility of body resistsnce. The scar or opacity resulting from inflammatory process of the cornea is called old nebula.

The membrane refers to the membranous tissue that extends from the limbus to the centre of the cornea. A membrane with a large number of new blood vessels or presenting as dartos is called red membrane (congestive pterygium), resulting from hyperactivity of wind heat in the liver and lung and from obstruction of the vessels. An uncongestive membrane is called white membrane and usually caused by excessive lung—Qi.

3.3 Differentiation of Common Signs of the Fundus

Optic disc: Congestion and edema of the disc with blurring margin are due to wind—heat of the liver channel or stagnation of the liver—Qi; pale disc and thin arteries are due to deficiency of the liver blood or deficiency of both *Qi* and blood. Papilledema is caused by stagnation of *Qi* and blood or insufficiency of *Yang* of both the spleen and kidney.

Vessels in the retina: Narrowed retinal arteries show hyperactivity of the liver—*Yang* or up-stirring of liver wind. If the retinal arteries become white and threadlike, it is due to wind phlegm which obstructs the vessels or due to upstirring of liver wind. Narrow retinal arteries and veins are due to deficiency of *Qi* and blood. Distended and tortuous retinal veins are due to stagnacy of *Qi* and blood stasis or are caused by flaring up of heart fire or hyperactivity of fire due to deficiency of *Yin*.

Macula retinae: Edema of macule retinae is due to dampness—heat retention and steaming within the body, or insufficiency of *Yang* of both the spleen and the kidney, or hyperactivity of fire due to deficiency of *Yin*. Hemorrhage in the region of macula is caused by failure of the spleen to keep the blood flowing within the blood vessels or by bleeding due to blood heat. Macula atrophy and degeneration are due to deficiency of both *Qi* and blood or deficiency of the liver and kidney.

Retina: Copious retinal hemorrhage with the blood in fresh scarlet color suggests abnormal flow of blood due to blood heat or hyperactivity of liver *Yang* or insufficiency of spleen *Qi*. Scanty retinal hemorrhage is caused by hyperactivity of fire due to deficiency of *Yin* or deficiency of *Qi* and blood.

Retinal edema is due to dysfunction of the spleen in transport or insufficiency of the kidney—*Yang,* retention of water in the body which leads to the upward motion of water, or stagnancy of *Qi* and blood stasis or retention, and steaming of dampness—heat.

Retinal exudation is usually caused by obstruction of lung-*Qi* or by retention of phlegm-dampness due to deficiency of *Yang* of the spleen and kidney, or by stagnation of liver-*Qi* and stagnancy of *Qi* and blood stasis.

Retinal retrograde degeneration is normally due to the consumption of *Qi* and blood or deficiency of the liver and kidney.

Vitreous: Vitreous inflammation opacity is due to the upward attack of turbid *Qi* or hyperactivity of fire due to deficiency of *Yin*. Hemorrhagic opacity is caused by stagnancy of *Qi* and blood stasis or by abnormal flow of blood due to blood heat or trauma.

In a word, all the pathologic changes of the tissues on the fundus are reflections of dysfunction of *Zang-Fu* organs. Hence in the course of differentiation of the diseases of the fundus overall analysis should be conducted according to the local manifestations combined with general symptoms. Only then can correct diagnosis be made.

4 The Essentials of Treatment

The eyes have close internal relationships with the *Zang-Fu* organs, channels, *Qi* and blood. Therefore, since ancient times, internal treatments have been taken as the principal methods for internal eye diseases, emphasizing differentiation of symptoms and signs on the holism and adapting oral administration of medicines. External eye diseases are treated with external therapeutic methods, directly applying medicines to the local affected area of the eye or performing surgical operations. Besides, acupuncture, moxibustion and massage are commonly used in ophthalmology.

4.1 Internal Treatment

On the basis of clinical differentiations, various therapies for internal treatment are established in accordance with the etiology and pathogenesis. Therapies of internal treatment often used in ophthalmology are naturally established in accordance with the common etiology and pathogenesis. Therapeutic methods are the basis for prescription, and prescription is realization of certain therapeutic methods. The basic principles of internal treatment in ophthalmology are similar to those in internal medicine, but they have some specific contents of their own. The common internal therapeutic methods used in ophthalmology are as follows.

Therapy of Dispelling Wind and Clearing Away Heat

Of all the eye diseases due to the attack of pathogenic wind and heat, the external oculopathy are most often seen. So the therapy of dispelling wind and clearing away heat is one of the common principles of treatment.

The symptoms of the attack of pathogenic wind and heat are redness, swelling and burning pain in the eye, photophobia and lacrimation, itching or profuse eye secretion. Sometimes they may be accompanied by general symptoms such as aversion to wind, fever, headache, floating and rapid pulse. In treatment, methods of dispelling wind are used to remove superficial symptoms; clearing away heat to remove heat syndromes.

Therapy of Purging Pathogenic Fire and Removing Toxic Material

It is a therapy in which medicines cold in nature are used so as to purge pathogenic fire and remove toxic materials. It is mainly used in eye diseases with symptoms of fire (heat) syndrome such as severe swelling of the eyelid, sore and carbuncle of the eyelid, hyperaemia of the bulbar conjunctiva, ulcer of the cornea, hypopyon, miosis etc. These symptoms are often accompanied with aching and tenderness, photophobia, lacrimation, and sometimes with such general symptoms as thirst, constipation, reddish tongue with yellowish fur.

This therapy is used very often in ophthalmology. Because of the difference in etiology and pathogenesis, the attack of pathogenic fire in the eye area must be carefully differentiated because it may be caused by liver fire, heart fire, lung fire, stomach fire of *San-Jiao* fire. Clinically this therapy must be used on the basis of differentiation of the symptoms and signs according to the state of the viscera. For example, for the cases with redness, swelling and burning pain of the eye, thirst and desire for drinking, constipation, the therapy of purging intense heat and inducing bowel movement should be used. For the cases with ciliary hyperaemia, nebula of the cornea, pain in the eyeball, yellow fur and wiry pulse, the therapy of clearing away liver fire should be adopted.

As this therapy tends to impair *Yang Qi* of the spleen and stomach of the patient, it can't be used for long, and the medicines with cooling nature must be carefully prescribed according to the patient's condition and constitution. Moreover, because of the cooling nature of the medicines, if this therapy is used too long, it will lead to stagnation of *Qi* and blood and the nebula will become difficult to remove. Therefore, for diseases of the cornea, this therapy must be used with great care. This therapy is contraindicated for the cases with fire of deficiency type.

Therapy of Nourishing *Yin* and Reducing Pathogenic Fire

By nourishing *Yin* and reducing fire of deficiency type, this therapy can relieve the symptoms of hyperactivity of pathogenic fire and *Yin* deficiency so as to improve visual ability. It is mainly used for the eye diseases due to *Yin* deficiency and hyperactivity of pathogenic fire. Fire of deficiency type due to consumption of *Yin* fluid flames up to attack the eye, causing slight redness and pain of the eye, thin eye secretion and tears, blurred vision. Sometimes these may be accompanied with dizziness, insomnia, dysphoria with feverish sensation in the chest, palms and soles, flushed cheeks, night sweat and nocturnal emission, cough with blood sputa, dysphoria and irritability, dry mouth and tongue, or tinitus and deafness, or retching and hiccup, or aphtha and erosion of the tongue, or low fever, red and dry tongue, little fur, thready and rapid pulse or feeble and rapid pulse.

Fire of deficiency type can further be subdivided into deficient fire of the heart, lung, stomach, liver and kidney. In clinical practice, medicine should be prescribed according to differentiation of symptoms and signs in association with the state of *Zang—Fu*. Symptoms such as macula or enkoma of cornea, slight ciliary, hyperaemia, dysphoria and irritability usually result from deficient fire of the liver channel; less blood vessels in both canthi, vexation and insomnia result from deficient fire of the heart channel; slight redness of the bulbar conjunctiva, dry nose and throat result from deficient fire of the lung channel, and pupillary metamorphosis, slight bleeding in the ocular fundus, tinitus and lumbago, dysphoria with feverish sensation in the chest, palms and soles result from deficient fire of kidney channel.

Therapy of Tonifying the Liver and Kidney

With the medicine of tonifying effect to the liver and kidney, this therapy can relieve the symptoms of consumption and deficiency of the liver and kidney and improve visual ability. The eye diseases of deficiency type mostly result from the deficiency of the liver and kidney. This therapy is indicated in such external eye diseases as hidden punctate nebula, rare and pale blood vessels of the bulbar conjunctiva and cold epiphora, as well as in such internal eye disorders as lustrelessness and blurred vision, myiodesopsia, optic atrophy and nyctalopia.

Meanwhile, whether the disease is due to deficiency of kidney—*Yin* or kidney—*Yang* it should be differentiated. For the cases with deficiency of kidney—*Yin*, tonifying kidney—*Yin* should be considered. For cases with deficiency of kidney—*Yang*, tonifying kidney—*Yang* should be prescribed. For cases with deficiency of *Yin* and *Yang*, tonify both.

Therapy of Benefiting *Qi* and Nourishing Blood

This therapy is to use medicines that have the nourishing effect to *Qi* and blood to relieve the symptoms of deficiency of *Qi* and blood so as to improve visual ability. In cases with deficiency of *Qi* and blood, the eye seems normal externally. There are such symptoms as lustreless eye, poor vision, or other visual abnormalities, or slight sensation of dryness and discomfort in the eye, slight hyperaemia of the bulbar conjunctiva.

Because *Qi* and blood depend on each other, benefiting *Qi* and nourishing blood are usually used at the same time. However, it must be determined which is more serious, deficiency of *Qi* or deficiency of blood, so that we can use this therapy flexibly. For instance, if the symptoms are tiredness, anorexia, eyelid ptosis, weakness in eye opening and closing, it can be ascertained that deficiency of *Qi* is more serious, so benefiting *Qi* is taken as the key. If the symptoms are poor vision, dizziness, palpitation and insomnia as a result of loss of blood or being ill for a long time, which usually result from blood deficiency, the therapy of nourishing blood should be considered.

As the spleen and stomach are organs that provide all essentials for life after one is born and transform *Qi* and blood from the foods and water after they are taken, in benefiting *Qi* and blood, They should be tonified too.

For cases with exuberant pathogens and without deficiency symptoms, this therapy can never be prescribed.

Therapy of Hemostasis

In this therapy the medicines used have a hemostatic effect to stop bleeding in the eye area. It is used for various symptoms of hemorrhage in the early stage, such as hemorrhage of the eyelid, subconjunctival ecchymosis, hyphema and intraocular hemorrhage.

Therapies for hemostasis vary with different causes of hemorrhage. For example, in the case of hemorrhage due to blood-heat, we should adopt the therapy of hemostasis by clearing away heat and cooling blood. When fire of deficiency type impairs the collaterals, we should adopt the therapy by tonifying *Yin* and removing heat from the blood. If it is caused by failure of controlling blood due to *Qi* deficiency, the therapy of benefiting *Qi* to control blood should be taken. For traumatic hemorrhage of the eye, hemostasis by removing blood stasis should be the key treatment.

This therapy is mainly used in the bleeding stage for emergency cases. If hemorrhage has stopped without the possibility of further bleeding, the therapy of activating blood circulation to remove blood stasis should gradually be used so as to promote absorption of stagnant blood and prevent residual of blood stasis.

Therapy of Activating Blood Circulation to Remove Blood Stasis

With the help of medicines that can activate blood circulation and remove blood stasis, this therapy can promote absorption of blood stasis in the eye. It is indicated for such disorders as hard, dark blue swelling of the eyelid, hemorrhage and ecchymosis of the bulbar conjunctiva, blood stasis in a certain part of the eye, stagnancy or obstruction of blood flow in the vessels of the retina, fixed pain in the eye, ecchymosis on the tongue, etc.

Qi is the motive force of blood flow and is responsible for the persistant circulation of blood. So in clinical practice, medicines with the property of activating *Qi* and removing stagnancy are often used compatibly with this therapy so as to improve the curative effect.

This therapy is contraindicated for pregnant women.

Therapy of Regulating *Qi*

This therapy includes nourishing *Qi* and activating *Qi*. The former is introduced in the Therapy of Benefiting *Qi* and Nourishing Blood, and this section only deals with the therapy of activating *Qi*.

By using medicines with dispersing and regulating effect, this therapy can improve pathologic conditions of dysfunction of viscera, channels and collaterals, obstruction of the functional activity of *Qi* so that it will raise the acuity of vision.

Depression and anger do harm to the liver and will result in dysfunction of dispersion of the liver and stagnation of liver—*Qi*, and this will cause many eye diseases, of which internal eye diseases including bluish glaucoma, green glaucoma and blurred vision occur most frequently. Both internal and external eye diseases with the symptoms of hypochondrial distention and fullness, depressed feeling in the chest, eructation, obstructed feeling in the pharynx, irritability and wiry pulse can be treated with therapy of dispersing the liver and regulating *Qi*.

Obstruction and stagnation of lung—*Qi* may also lead to eye diseases such as hemorrhage of the bulbar conjunctiva, edema in the eye area, accompanied with the symptom of impeded cough. The proper therapy for this case is activating *Qi* and promoting flow of lung—*Qi*.

For the eye diseases due to dysfunction of the spleen and stomach, dyspepsia, stagnation of *Qi*, the therapy of activating *Qi* and removing stagnation and retention can be used. In addition, if the patient has symptoms of blood stasis in the eye, medicines with the effect of activating blood circulation and removing blood stasis should be used compatibly.

For cases suffering from deficiency of *Qi* and *Yin,* this therapy should be adopted with great care.

Therapy of Dispelling Dampness

This therapy is to use medicines with the effect of dispelling pathogenic dampness to treat eye diseases. It is indicated for diseases of the eyes due to the retention of water in the viscera and channels, such as edema of the eyelid, ulcerative marginal blepharitis, miliaria in the eyelid, xanthosis of the bulbar conjunctiva, gnawed opacity of the cornea, interstitial keratitis, vitrous opacity and blurred vision, possibly accompanied with clamped headache, no thirst or thirst without desire of drinking, depression in the chest, poor appetite, abdominal distention and loose stools, myasthenia of the limbs, or cough with sputa, etc.

As the positions invaded by pathogenic dampness and the accompanying pathogenic factors are different, the therapeutic methods actually adopted are also different. For instance, a wet and itching eyelid caused by invasions of wind and dampness can be treated with therapy of dispelling wind—dampness. Diseases caused by upward assault of dampness—heat such as marginal blepharitis, alternative attack of wet and itching on the eyelid, ulceration of the cornea can be treated by clearing away the dampness—heat. Cases with the stagnation of phlegm—dampness have painful swelling on the eyelid, or blurred vision and muscaegenetic vision, and retinal edema, group and petechial exudation on the retina and choroid in ocular fundus examination. They may also have whitish and greasy fur and slow pulse. The therapy of removing phlegm—dampness should then be considered. The therapy of removing dampness and promoting diuresis can be used for retinal edema caused by floating up of dampness. Cold and deficiency syndromes of middle—*Jiao* with stagnation of dampness may lead to blurred vision, chromatopsia, accompanied with dizziness, heavy and weary sensation in the limbs, cold limbs, pale tongue with smooth fur, deep and slow pulse. These can be treated with the therapy of warming the middle—*Jiao* to dispel cold and activating *Yang* to promote diuresis.

Therapy of Removing Nebula to Improve Vision

This therapy can improve the acuity of vision by prescribing medicines with the power of removing the nebula. It is a unique therapy in TCM ophthalmology, and is indicated for punctate nebula on the diseased cornea.

However, the therapy of removing the nebula must be practised by steps. For instance, at the onset of the disease which is marked by punctate nebula, redness and lacrimatiom, there exists intense wind—heat, and the chief therap should be dispelling wind and clearing away heat; besides, proper medicines for removing nebula can be added if necessary. When the wind—heat is gradually reduced, we can add more medicines for removing nebula on the basis of the therapy above. In the late stage of the disease, the wind heat has been completely cleared away, but the nebula still remains, with deficiency of vital—*Qi*, nebula—removing medicines should be mainly considered, though some medicines for benefiting *Qi* and blood or nourishing the liver and kidney are also necessary. Because the black of the eye is closely related to the liver, medicines with the property of clearing away liver—heat, calming the liver and dispersing stagnant liver—Qi also have the effect of removing the nebula and so can be used in this therapy. In the late stage when medicines for removing nebula form the main part of the prescription, the property of the medicines can not be too cold, lest the effects may impair vital—Qi, leading to incubation of pathogenic factors, stagnation of Qi and blood, which makes it difficult to remove the nebula.

4.2 External Treatment

Widely used in clinical practice, external treatment of eye diseases has been one of the main therapies in TCM ophthalmology since the ancient dynasties. Therapies to use medicines directly to the eye or the area near the eye are known as external treatment. It may be adopted in combination with internal treatment, especially for external eye diseases. In treating quite a few internal eye diseases such as bluish glaucoma, miosis, cataract, etc, internal treatment should be considered with external treatment. Therefore, external treatment is an indispensable link in treating eye diseases.

There are many types of external treatment. Besides dropping, fumigation and washing, topical application and fomentation with heated drugs, some surgical methods like hooking, cutting, cauterization and needling treatment are considered to be of great importance. Modern TCM ophthalmology has not only carried forward traditional external treatments but also improved them actively. The commonly—used external treatments are as follows.

1. Therapy of Dropping

Being one of the external treatments often used in TCM ophthalmology, this therapy is to drop medicines directly into the eye. It is indicated for ulceration of the eyelid, hyperaemia of the bulbar conjunctiva, swelling and itching, blood vessels spreading over the eyes, membrane corneal ulceration and nebula, constriction and pupillary metamorphosis due to posterior synechia, five-coloured glaucoma, cataract at the early stage. In clinical practice, the usual preparations include eye drops, eye ointment and eye powder.

2. Therapy of Fumigation and Washing

As a traditional curative method, this therapy is to use the uprising steam of the boiled medicines to heat the affected area. After fumigation, filter the decoction and use it to wash the affected area. In general, fumigate the affected area first, then wash it, or only fumigate it. Besides the effect of wet-hot compresses, this therapy can dredge the channels, remove wind and clear away heat, eliminate toxic substances and promote detumescence through the direct action of various drugs on the eye. It is mainly used for the external eye diseases such as swelling eyelid, photophobia, dryness and pain, profuse eye secretion and tears.

3. Therapy of Application

(1) Hot-application

Hot-application can dredge the channels, activate Qi and blood, remove blood stasis, promote detumescence and alleviate pain. It is adoptable for external eye diseases with conjunctival congestion, swelling and pain, blood stasis and swelling of the eyelid, bulbar conjunctival hemorrhage by trauma for 24 hours, and nonfresh hemorrhagic pupil.

This therapy is contraindicated for cases with pyogenesis as localized focus and fresh hemorrhage of the affected eye.

(2) Cold-application

Cold-application has the effect of clearing away heat to relieve pain, cooling the blood to stop bleeding. It is indicated for subcutaneous hemorrhage of eyelid trauma in the early stage, or burning swelling pain in the eye. An ice bag or a towel soaked in cold water is usually applied to the eye.

(3) Topical Application with Drugs

Some medicines have the property of cooling blood to stop bleeding, clearing away heat and toxic materials, removing blood stasis, promoting detumescence and relieving pain, dispelling wind and alleviating itching. In this therapy, these medicines are often selected and applied topically to the eyelid for various external eye diseases and trauma.

4. Therapy of Irrigation

Generally speaking, this method refers to the irrigation of the conjunctival sac and lacrimal passage. It is used for the conjunctival diseases with the symptoms of profuse secretion and tear, the splash of chemical fluid into the eye, or foreign bodies in the conjunctival sac and the clearing of the conjunctival sac before a surgical operation. It can also be used to examine whether the lacrimal passage is free from obstruction and to remove the secretion accumulated in the lacrimal sac, or used as a routine preparation for an intra-ocular operation.

5. Therapy of Hooking and Cutting

As a common surgicad in TCM ophthalmology, this therapy is used to relieve the symptoms of pterygium and vegetation in the eye. During the operation, pierce the pterygium with a sharp needle, pull it up, then gradually separate it from the cornea and the conjunctiva with a hoe-knife and cut the pterygium away. It must be done with slight motions and the tissues must be separated completely. After the removal, cauterize the area to prevent recurrence. The process is more or less similar to that of cutting pterygium in Western Medicine.

6. Therapy of Cauterization

This therapy is to put the specially-made cauterizing apparatus on the fire till it becomes red and hot. Then cauterize the affected part of the eye. It is used often after hooking and cutting, so as to prevent recurrence and stop bleeding in a surgical operation. Also it can be used for chronic blepharitis marginalis. During cauterization, special attention should be paid to protection of the healthy tissues such as the eyelid, canthus, the cornea, etc. The temperature of cauterization should not be too high, lest the deeper tissues should be burned and injured.

7. Therapy of Needle-puncture

This therapy is prescribed to remove cataract. There are three types of needles used in clinical practice: three-edged needles, sword-like needles and metal needles.

(1) Three-edged Needle Treatment

This treatment is to puncture a certain point to cause bleeding with a three-edged needle; or it is used in sickle therapy to puncture and scrape the accumulated granules in the affected area. With the function of removing blood stasis and stagnation, it can be used for external eye diseases of excess syndrome with the symptoms of redness, heat and swelling.

(2) Swordlike Needle Treatment

This type of needle, with a double edge and a sharp point like that of a sward can be used for piercing and cutting. It is used to cut away pterygium and other vegetations in the eye area, to pierce and incise pustulous sore, to remove foreign bodies imbedded in the bulbar conjunctiva and cornea.

(3) Metal Needle Treatment for Removing Cataract

This is an important surgical method in treating round cataract in TCM ophthalmology. It can be used for mature round cataract in the elderly. On the basis of this traditional therapy, modern TCM doctors have assimilated the merits of the similar operation in Western Medicine, and created the therapy of removing cataract with the combination of TCM and Western Medicine.

Method: When operating on the left eye for example, the surgeon sits in front of the patient on the side of the eye to be operated on. The assistant stands behind the patient. Sutures are made to tow the lower eyelid. The assistant pulls up the upper eyelid with a pulling hook.

Incision: The surgeon obtains a grasp of the conjunctiva tissues near the corneal margin at 6 o'clock meridian with a fixation forceps and draws the eyeball, turning it to the nasal side. A triangular blade is thrust into the point 4 mm. outward the corneal margin at 4—5 o' clock meridian, perforates the wall of the eyeball vertically, makes a 3 mm. long incision parallel to the corneal margin.

Couching: The sequence of cutting off the suspensory ligament of the lens is as follows:

① Cutting of the 4—5 o' clock ligament. The couching needle is held with the concave facing downwards. After the needle has been inserted vertically into the incision for a depth of about 3 mm. the head of the needle is directed to 12 o' clock meridian and the needle is pushed forward slightly and swingingly between the ciliary body and the lens. On reaching the pupillar margin at 12 o′ clock meridian, the concave of the needle is kept close to the lens, bypasses the equator, under beneath, cut off the 4—6 o′ clock suspensory ligament.

② Cutting of the supertemporal ligament. After the needle is directed behind and beneath the lens, the head of the needle is levelled. By small lateral movements of the needle at about one third of the pupillary zone from the nasal side to the temporal side, the front vitreous membrane is cut. Then the needle is rotated with the concave facing downwards, withdrawn about one half, reinserted to the front of the lens near the equator at 1—4 o′ clock. The lens is pressed backwards and downwards.

③ Cutting of the super nasal suspensory ligament. The head of the needle is introduced to the front of the lens at 9—10 o′ clock meridian. A pressure is made to press the lens backwards and downwards to rupture the 9—10 o′ clock suspersory ligament. When the lens stays horizontally, another division is made on the front vitreous membrane by the needle.

④ Cutting of the inferior nasal suspensory ligament to finish the couching. The concave of the needle should get hold of the lens on the superior nasal side at the 9—10 o′ clock equator, turning the 12 o′ clock to the intraocular subtemporal side at pars plana corporis ciliaris and ora serrata retinae. The suspensory ligament at about 6 o′ clock should not be cut.

Withdrawal of the needle: When the lens does not float after the needle is lifted, the needle can be withdrawn. The conjunctival incision is adjusted to make it cover the incision of the sclera. Hormone and antibiotic can be injected under the conjunctiva.

Mydriasis and a monocular dressing are applied.

Caution: When the needle is inserted into the incision with a sensation of resistance, the following factors should be considered: The incision is too small, or the pars plana corporis ciliaris is not cut through, or there is entrance of the retinal tissues into the incision. In cutting off the subtemporal ligament, as the needle passes the equator beneath the lens, it should not be directed beyond the 6 o′ clock too much lest the ligament at 6 o′ clock be cut off. Otherwise, after the operation the lens will be in a free state and will move with changes of the body position to influence the vision in the upper field. When cutting the front retreous membrane, the needle should not get into the eye too much, lest it should damage the ciliary body or the ora serrata retinae.

4.3 Common Medicines of Ophthalmology

Oral Medicines

1. Medicines for Removing Wind

Wind, the primary pathogen, is apt to change. It often causes diseases in association with heat, cold, damp by attacking the channels, collaterals and *Zang-Fu*. The eyes are at the upper part of the body and apt to be attacked by pathogenic wind. Therefore, wind-removing medicines are used commonly in ophthalmology. Because the property of wind-removing medicines is pungent with dissipating effects, which tends to impair *Yin* and body fluids, these medicines should be used cautiously for patients with excess of Yang and flaring up of fire, hyperactive internal heat, *Yin* and blood deficiency, deficiency-syndrome of superficies with hyperhidrosis. For patients affected by endogenous wind, these medicines cannot be taken without care.

Wind-removing medicines have the effects of removing wind promoting detumescence, alleviating pain and itching. They are mostly indicated for early external eye diseases with the symptoms of redness, swelling and pain in the eye, stabbing itching, lacrimation and punctate nebula at the early stage. There are two categories of these commonly used medicines: medicines of dispelling pathogens in the superficies with acrid taste and cool property, medicines of dispelling pathogens in the superficies with acrid taste and warm property.

(1) Medicines of dispelling pathogens in the superficies with acrid taste and cool property.

The commonly used medicines are Folium Mori, Flos Chrysanthemi, Radix Bupleuri, Herba Menthae, Fructus Viticis, Radix Puerariae, Periostracum Cicadae, etc. Folium Mori and Flos Chrysanthemi have the effects of dispelling wind and heat, clearing away liver fire to improve vision. In treating eye diseases due to wind-heat of the liver channel, they are often used logether. Radix Bupleuri has the effect of removing heat, dispersing stagnant liver-*Qi*, removing nebula and lifting up *Qi* of the middle warmer. By different compatibility with other medicines, it can be used extensively for various kinds of internal and external eye diseases such as corneal nebula, greenish glaucoma, miosis due to wind-heat and liver-heat, and blephariptosis, optic atrophy due to deficiency of middle warmer *Qi*. Radix Puerariae can dispel pathogens in the superficies of *Yangming*, and it is often used to treat the eye diseases due to wind-heat, accompanied with pain in the forehead. Periostracum Cicadae can remove wind—heat, improve vision, remove nebula and alleviate itching. It is often administered to treat corneal nebula, blepharitis marginalis, trachoma, miliary eruptions with gargalesthetic sensation in the eye. The typical prescription is *Yin Qiao San*.

(2) Medicines of dispelling pathogens in the superficies with acrid taste and warm property.

Medicines of this category in common use include Herba Schizonepetae, Radix Ledebouriellae, Rhizoma seu Radix Notopterygii, Radix Angelicae Dahuricae, Radix Angelicae Pubescentis, Herba Asari, Rhizoma Ligustici, etc. Among them, Herba Schizonepetae, Radix Ledebouriellae and Rhizoma seu Radix Notopterygii have strong effects of dispelling wind, alleviating pain and itching, and removing nebula. The three medicines can be used together for ciliary hyperemia, nebula, pain in the eye and head, intense itching due to exogenous wind and cold, and, of the three, Rhizoma seu Radix Notopterygii has a stronger effect of dispelling wind—damp, and can be used for eye diseases and headache due to wind—damp and wind—cold. Herba Schizonepetae has a slight effect of removing heat, and can treat blood disorders and sores. Radix Ledebouriellae has an effect of activating the channels and removing substantial masses and blood stasis. It is often used compatibly with drugs of activating blood flow in treatment of miliary eruptions, acute scleritis due to stagnation of blood and *Qi*, and pain due to blood stasis after a trauma or an operation. Rhizoma Ligustici can be used to treat pain in the eye accompanied with *Taiyang* parietal headache.

The typical prescription is Qufeng Yizi San.

2. Medicines for clearing away heat

At the position of lucid *Yang* and as an orifice to the liver, the eye is susceptive to pathogenic heat and flaming-up of liver fire. So the eye diseases with heat-syndrome are often seen. Medicines for clearing away heat have cool and cold property, and so are used for all kinds of eye diseases with heat-syndrome due to flaming-up heat and fire.

According to their specific properties, these medicines can be divided into heat-clearing and fire-eliminating drugs, heat-clearing and detoxifying drugs, heat-clearing and purging drugs, heat-clearing and vision-improving drugs, etc.

As these medicines are cool and cold in property, they tend to impair *Yang-Qi*. So they should be used carefully for patients with deficiency of *Yang-Qi*, deficiency and cold of the spleen and stomach, loose stools. If the drugs bitter in taste and cold in property are taken for a long time, it will easily cause impairment of *Yin* and resultant dryness. Therefore, for the patient with deficiency of *Yin*, these medicines should be prescribed with great care.

(1) Medicines for heat-clearing and fire-eliminating

These medicines are used to treat eye diseases owing to the accumulation of heat and fire of excess type. The commonly-used are Gypsum Fibrosum, Rhizoma Anemarrhenae, Fructus Gardeniae, Cortex Mori Radicis, Rhizoma Coptidis, Radix Scutellariae, Cortex Phellodendri, Herba Lophatheri, Radix Gentianae, etc. Among them, Rhizoma Coptidis and Herba Lophatheri can purge heart fire, relieve vexation, and are often prescribed for patients with canthitis. Radix Scutellariae and Cortex Mori Radicis can purge lung fire, and are mainly used to treat conjunctival hyperemia. Gypsum Fibrosum and Rhizoma Anemarrhenae can purge stomach fire, and are used to treat redness and swelling of the eyelid, hypopyon. Fructus

Gardeniae can purge *San-Jiao* fire. When it is used compatibly with other heat-clearing drugs, various eye diseases due to heat of excess type can be treated. Radix Gendianae can purge the fire of excess type in the liver and gallbadder, and is often used to treat corneal diseases due to flaming-up of liver fire. Cortex Phellodendri and Rhizoma Anemarrhenae can purge kidney fire and remove fire of deficiency type. Used compatibly with Rhizoma Coptidis and Radix Scutellariae, they can treat eye diseases due to dampness-heat.

The typical prescriptions are *Xie Xin Tang*, *Xie Fei Tang*, *Tong Pi Xie Wei Tang* and *Long Dan Xie Gan Tang*.

(2) Medicines for heat-clearing and detoxifying

These medicines are used to treat all kinds of eye diseases of excess-heat type due to pathogenic fire, heat and toxic materials. The commonly used are: Flos Lonicerae, Fructus Forsythiae, Flos Chrysanthmi, Folium Isatidis, Radix Isatidis, Herba Taraxaci, Herba Violae, etc. Eye diseases caused by pathogenic fire vary, so in most cases, these drugs should be used with others according to the patient's condition. For example, drugs for dispelling pathogenic wind such as Rhizoma Cimicifugae, Radix Ledebouriellae and Herba Schizonepetae should be added to the prescription for patients with pathogenic factors attacking the exterior of the body. For patients with redness, swelling and burning pain in the eye, drugs for clearing heat, cooling blood, activating blood and alleviating pain should be added, such as Cortex Moutan Radicis, Radix Paeoniae Rubra, Radix et Rhizoma Rhei, Resina Boswelliae Carterii, Resina Commiphorae Myrrhae, etc. For patients suffering from sore and carbuncle on the eye area with suppuration and difficult to rupture, Squama Manitis and Spina Gleditsiae should be added to expel toxins and drain the pus.

The typical prescription is *Qingre Jiedu Tang*

(3) Medicines for clearing away heat through purgation

These medicines are used to treat eye diseases with the symptoms of redness, swelling and pain of the eye, sticky eye secretion accompanied with constipation due to excess syndrome of *Yang-ming* hollow organs, flaming-up of the interior fire. The commonly used are Radix et Rhizoma Rhei, Natrii Sulfas, etc.

The typical prescription is *Dacheng Qi Tang*

(4) Medicines for clearing away heat and cooling blood

These drugs are used to treat eye diseases due to invasion of pathogenic heat into the blood and *Ying*. The commonly used include Cornu Rhinoceri, Radix Scrophulariae, Radix Rehmanniae, Cortex Moutan Radicis, Radix Paeoniae Rubra, Radix Arnebiae seu Lithospermi, etc.

Among them, Cornu Rhinoceri and Radix Arnebiae seu Liyhospermi can cool blood and remove toxic materials, and are often used to treat hemorrhage and sudden diminution of vision due to hyperactivity of blood heat caused by abundant heat pathogen. Cortex Moutan Radicis and Radix Paeoniae Rubra can clear away heat, cool and activate blood and remove blood stasis, and are used to treat eye diseases due to stagnant heat in the blood system. With the effect of clearing away heat, cooling blood, nourishing *Yin* and promoting the production of body fluid, Radix Rehmanniae and Radix Scrophulariae are indicated for eye diseases in association with hemorrhage due to blood-heat, deficiency of *Yin* and inadequacy of body fluids.

The typical prescription is *Qingying Tang*

(5) Medicines of clearing away heat to improve vision

These medicines are mainly used to treat punctate nebula due to wind—heat. The commonly used include Spica Prunellae, Semen Cassiae, Semen Celosiae, Flos Buddlejae, Herba Equiseti Hiemalis, etc. Spica Prunellae can eliminate the stagnant fire of the liver and gallbadder, and is often used to treat eye diseases with the symptoms of redness, swelling and pain of the eye, and hemorrhage in the ocular fundus due to liver fire. Semen Cassiae and Semen Celosiae can clear away liver fire and improve visual ability. Flos Buddlejae can dispel wind—heat and remove conjunctival congestion, nourish the liver and moisten dryness. Herba Equiseti Hiemalis can dispel wind and clear away heat, remove nebula to improve visual ability.

The typical prescription is *Shijueming San*.

3. Medicines for Invigoration

Eye diseases of the type of deficiency syndrome mostly result from deficiency of *Qi* and blood, or from insufficiency of the liver and kidney. So among medicines for invigoration, those with the property of replenishing *Qi* and blood and nourishing the liver and kidney are used commonly.

(1) Medicines for nourishing *Qi* and blood

These medicines are used to treat blepharochalasis, excavational nebula and optic atrophy due to deficiency of *Qi*. The commonly used include Radix Astragali seu Hedysari, Radix Ginseng, Rhizoma Atractylodis Macrocephalae, Rhizoma Dioscoreae and Radix Glycyrrhizae. Medicines that can nourish blood are used for patients with dryness sensation, discomfort of the eye and blurred vision, night blindness and optic atrophy due to deficiency of blood. The following are frequently prescribed: Rhizoma Rehmanniae Praeparatae, Radix Angelicae Sinensis,

Radix Paeoniae Alba, Radix Polygoni Multiflori, Colla Corii Asini and Fructus Mori.

The typical prescription of medicines for nourishing *Qi* is *Buzhong Yiqi Tang* and the typical prescription of medicines for nourishing blood is *Siwu Tang*.

(2) Medicines for nourishing the liver and kidney.

These medicines are used to treat both internal and external eye diseases due to insufficiency of the liver and kidney. They can be divided into two categories: medicines for nourishing the liver and kidney, medicines for warming and recuperating kidney—*Yang*. Medicines for nourishing the liver and kidney in common use include Rhizoma Rehmanniae Praeparatae, Fructus Lycii, Fructus Rubi, Fructus Ligustri Lucidi, Fructus Tribuli, Semen Astragali Complanati, Semen Cuscutae, Fructus Broussonetiae, etc. Among them, Rhizoma Rehmanniae Praeparatae has stronger effect of nourishing *Yin*, so it is the first to be selected for internal eye diseases due to *Yin* deficiency. Fructus Lycii has the effect of nourishing the liver and kidney, replenishing refined energy to improve vision. So it is widely used often compatibly with Flos Chrysanthemi to treat internal and external eye diseases due to deficiency of the liver and kidney. Fructus Ligustri Lucidi can nourish kidney—*Yin*, and treat *Yin* deficiency and internal heat. In management of hemorrhage in the eye at the early stage, it is often used compatibly with Herba Ecliptae which has the effect of nourishing kidney—*Yin*, cooling blood and stopping bleeding. Fructus Rubi can nourish the liver and kidney, strengthen refined energy to improve vision. Both Semen Astragali Complanati and Semen Cuscutae can nourish the kidney, replenish refined energy to improve vision. Fructus

Broussonetiae can calm and recuperate the liver and kidney, nourish the liver to improve visual ability.

To warm and recuperate kidney—*Yang*, the medicines in common use include Placenta Hominis, Cornu Cervi Pantotrichum, Radix Morindae officinalis, Herba Epimedii, Fructus Psoraleae, Cortex Cinnamomi, Radix Aconiti Praeparata, etc.

The typical prescriptions are *Liuwei Dihuang Wan* and *Yougui Wan*.

4. Medicines for treating blood disorders.

These medicines are mainly used to treat pathogenic changes of the blood system such as hemorrhage, blood stasis, blood heat and blood deficiency which should be treated respectively by stopping bleeding, activating blood circulation to remove blood stasis, cooling blood and nourishing blood. The latter two therapies have been discussed in the sections of Medicines for clearing heat and medicines for invigoration.

(1) Medicines for stopping bleeding

These drugs can be used to treat all kinds of hemorrhage in the eye at the bleeding stage. According to the pathogenesis and properties of hemorrhage, their effect of bleeding—arrest can be sorted as hemostasis by cooling blood, hemostasis by astringency, hemostasis by warming channels and hemostasis by removing blood stasis.

Medicines with hemostasic effect by cooling blood are used to treat hemorrhagic symptoms of the eye due to abnormal flow caused by blood heat at the bleeding stage. The commonly used are Herba seu Radix Cirsii Japonici, Herba Cephalanoploris, Radix Sanguisorbae, Rhizoma Imperatae, Herba Ecliptae, etc.

Medicines with hemostasic effect by astringency are used for fresh hemorrhage in all kinds of eye diseases and ocular trauma before blood stasis is formed. The drugs in common use include Herba Agrimoniae, Rhizoma Bletillae, Nodus Nelumbinis Rhizomatis, Crinis Cerbonisatus, Fuligo Plantae, etc. Medicines with hemostasic effect by warming channels are used to treat hemorrhage of cold-syndrome. The commonly used are Folium Artemisiae Argyi, Terraflava Usta, Herba Schizonepetae. Medicines with hemostasic effect by removing blood stasis are used to treat hemorrhage due to obstruction by blood stasis. These medicines have the effect of stopping bleeding and removing blood stasis. The commonly used are Radix Notoginseng, Pollen Typhae, Resina Draconis, Ophicalcitum, Radix Rubiae, etc.

The typical prescription is *Shihui San*.

(2) Medicines for activating blood circulation to remove blood stasis.

These medicines are used for cases with blood stasis in the eye after hemostasis, or with eye diseases due to obstruction of blood stasis. The commonly used are: Semen Persicae, Flos Carthami, Herba Lycopi, Rhizoma Ligustici Chuanxiong, Radix Salviae Miltiorrhizae, Herba Artemisiae Anomalae, Semen Vaccariae, Radix Achyranthis Bidentatae, Radix Paeoniae Rubra, Cortex Moutan Radicis, Resina Boswelliae Carterii, Resina Commiphorae Myrrhae, Faeces Trogopterorum, Lignum Sappan, Hirudo, Tabanus Bivittatus, etc.

The typical prescription is *Xuefu Zhuyu Tang*.

5. Medicines for regulating *Qi*

Regulating *Qi* is a therapeutic method of putting in order the flow of *Qi*. All the eye diseases due to disorder of *Qi* can be treated with the medicines that can regulate *Qi*. However, these medicines are mostly acrid, warm and diaphoretic, which tend to consume *Qi* and impair *Yin*. So for patients with *Yin* insufficiency, they should be used carefully.

Qi-regulating medicinces commonly used in ophthalmology can be divided into three categories: medicines for dispersing stagnant liver-*Qi*, medicines for activating *Qi* to benefit the lung, medicines for activating *Qi* to remove stagnancy.

(1) Medicines for dispersing stagnant liver-*Qi*.

These medicines are often used to treat the internal eye diseases due to depressed emotion and stagnation of liver-*Qi*, such as greenish glaucoma, bluish glaucoma, blurred vision, vitreous opacity, optic atrophy, sudden loss of vision. The commonly used include Radix Bupleuri, Pericarpium Citri Reticulatae Viride, Rhizoma Cyperi, Radix Curcumae, Rhizoma Ligustici Chuanxiong, Fructus Meliae Tosendan, etc.

The typical prescription is *Xiaoyao San*.

(2) Medicines for activating *Qi* to benefit the lung.

These medicines are used to treat hyperemia of the bulbar conjunctiva, or severe swelling, or subjunctival echymosis due to obstruction of *Qi* flow resulting from failure of the lung-*Qi* to descend. The commonly used include Cortex Mori Radicis, Radix Platycodi, Radix Peucedani, Flos Inulae, Fructus Perillae, Semen Armeniacae Amarum, Cortex Lycii Radicis, Folium Eriobotryae, etc.

The typical prescription is *Xie bai San*.

(3) Medicines for activating *Qi* to remove stagnancy.

These medicines are used to treat redness and swelling of the eyelid, itching, pain and furuncle on the eye area, or eye disorder due to malnutrition in children, or blurred vision caused by disorder of the spleen and stomach, interior indigestion and stagnation. The commonly used are Fructus Aurantii Immaturus, Pericarpium Citri Reticulatae, Cortex Magnoliae Officinalis, Radix Aucklandiae, Fructus Amomi, Lignum Aquilariae Resinatum, Semen Raphani, Semen Arecae, etc, and they are often used compatibly with medicines for relieving dyspepsia such as Fructus Crataegi, Massa Fermentata Medicinalis, Endothelium Corneum Gigeriae Galli, etc.

The typical prescription is *Baohe Wan*.

6. Medicines for removing dampness.

Medicines for removing dampness are used to treat eye diseases due to pathogenic dampness. These medicines can be divided into sevsral types: aromatics that can remove dampness, diuretics that can promote discharge of dampness, tastless drugs that can excrete dampness, bitter-tasted and cold-property drugs that can dry dampness, *Yang*-warming drugs that can excrete dampness. Among them, aromatics that can remove dampness and diuretics that can excrete dampness are used more frequently in ophthalmology.

(1) Aromatics that can remove dampness.

These are used to treat eye diseases due to interior obstruction and stagnation of pathogenic dampness. The commonly used include Herba Agastachis, Herba Eupatorii, Rhzioma Atractylodis, Fructus Amomi, Semen Cardamoni Rotundi, Rhizoma Acori Graminei, etc.

The typical prescription is *Huoxiang Zhengqi San*.

(2) Diuretics that can excrete dampness.

These are used to treat eye diseases caused by retention of

water and dampness in the body. The commonly used are Poria, Polyporus Umbellatus, Semen Plantaginis, Rhizoma Alismatis, Talcum, Semen Coicis, Semen Phaseoli, etc.

The typical prescription is *Wuling San*.

7. Medicines for eliminating phlegm to resolve substantial masses.

These can be used to treat eye diseases due to phlegm, such as subcutaneous nodule of the eyelid, edema of the ocular fundus by the accumulation of phlegm in the eye, profuse secretion, ocular tumour, exophthalmus, etc. The commonly used consist of two major types: medicines of eliminating phlegm by warming up cold, medicines of eliminating phlegm by clearing away heat. The former often includes Rhizoma Pinelliae, Rhizoma Arisaematis, Semen Sinapis Albae, Fructus Gleditsiae Abnoumalis, Flos Inulae, etc. And the latter often includes Fructus Trichosanthis, Bulbus Fritillariae, Semen Lepiddii seu Descurainiae, Lapis Chloriti, Os Costaziae, Thallus Laminariae, Sargassum, etc.

The typical prescriptions are *Erchen Tang* and *Qingtan Yin*.

8. Medicines for removing nebula to improve vision.

These medicines are used to treat corneal nebula shortly after recession of pathogenic *Qi*. In general, medicines that can dispell wind—heat or medicines that can clear away liver—heat and calm the liver have the effect of removing nebula, The commonly used are : Periostracum Cicadae, Cortex Fraxini, Flos Eriocauli, Herba Equiseti Hiemalis, Flos Buddejae, Concha Haliotidis, Concha Margaritifera Usta, Fructus Tribuli, Semen Celosiae, Periostracum Serpentis, etc.

Among them, Perioatracum Cicadae, Cortex Fraxini, Flos Eriocauli and Flos Buddlejae can remove nebula caused by wind-heat. and Concha Haliotidis, Concha Margaritifera Usta, Fructus Tribuli and Semen Celosiae can remove nebula due to liver-heat. Medicines for removing nebula are mostly demulcent, and can be used compatibly with other kinds of medicines in treatment of new and old nebula.

The typical prescription is *Shijueming San*.

Common medicines for external use in ophthalmology include

1. Mineral medicines: Realgar, Cinnabaris, Calamina, Borax, Sal Ammoniaci, Achates, Fossilia Brachyurae, Fossilia Spiriferis, etc.

2. Medicines from animals: Fel Ursi, Fel Sus Scrofa Domestuca Brisson, Fel Capra Hircus L, Fel Mylophartngodon Puceys, Moschus, Calculus Bovis, Os Sepoae, Periostracum Cicadae, Periostracum Serpentis, Concha Haliotidis, Concha Margaritifera Usta, etc.

3. Herbal medicines: Flos Lonicerae, Herba Taraxaci, Rhizoma Coptidis, Radix Scutellariae, Cortex Phellodendri, Indigo Naturalis, Radix Gentianae, Radix Arnebiae seu Lithospermi, Radix Rehmanniae, Flos Chrysanthemi, Herba Menthae, Herba Equiseti Hiemalis, Herba Schizonepetae, Radix Ledebouriellae, Cormus Eleocharis, Radix Notoginseng, Resina Commiphorae Mrrhae, Resina Boswelliae Carterii, etc. According to their properties, these medicines can be made into such preparations for external use as water solution, ointment, powder, lozenge, membrane, etc.

5 Diseases of the Eyelids

The eyelids are termed as *Baojian* or *Yanbi* in TCM. They are classified as flesh orbiculus in the five orbiculi which corresponds to the spleen. The spleen and the stomach are interior–exteriorly related. Therefore diseases of the eyelids have a close relationship with the spleen and the stomach. For example, improper diet or taking too much purgent, fried foods may bring about dysfunction of the spleen and stomach, causing retention of dampness–heat in the interior which will further convert into fire and go up to attack the eye, and so diseases of the eyelid will occur. Poor nourishment of eyelid resulting from sinking of *Qi* of middle–*Jiao*, deficiency of both *Qi* and blood may also induce such diseases. Eyelids are the outer–most part of the eyes, so they are apt to be attacked by external pathogenic wind and other noxious agents. The onset of the disease is sudden with marked local symptoms. Therefore, in analysis of the case, both local and general symptoms should be taken into consideration so as to determine that the disease is caused by exopathogen or by internal injury. For diseases caused by exogenous wind–heat, the treatment is mainly to dispel wind and to clear away heat and toxic materials. For diseases caused by fire or heat in the spleen and stomach, the therapy is to clear away heat and eliminate the toxic materials. For diseases caused by retention of dampness–heat in the interior, it is to clear away heat and promote diuresis. For diseases caused by combined attack of exogenous evils and endogenous pathogens, both internal and external treatment should be used.

5.1 Hordeolum

Hordeolum is an acute suppurative inflammation of the eyelid glands (sebaceous gland, palpebral glands). It is mainly caused by staphylococci. According to the affected position, hordeolum is classified into two types: the internal hordeolum and the external hordeolum. This disease is termed as *Zhenyan* in TCM, also known as *Tu Gan* and *Tu Yang*.

Etiology and Pathogenesis

The disease is usually caused by stagnation of *Qi* and blood in the eyelids as a result of invasion by wind—heat pathogen, or , by injury to the eyes from accumulation of pathogenic heat in the spleen and stomach due to over—intake of pungent or fried foods.

Clinical Manifestations

At the early stage, there is pain in the eyelids which is followed by local swelling and redness. Nodule may be palpated with tenderness. In the case of external hordeolum a yellow or yellowish pustule is formed at the part of the eyelash roots. In an internal hordeolum the yellow pustule is seen on the surface of the palpebral conjunctiva. At the outer canthus, hyperemia of bulbar conjunctiva and edema may appear. In severe cases, there may be swollen lymphoglandulaes auriculares anteriores with tenderness.

Type and Treatment

1. Internal Treatment

(1) Type of attack of pathogenic wind—heat.

Symptoms and Signs: The patient feels as if there were

something foreign in the affected eye, which suffers from exposure to wind, slight pain and photophobia, slight swelling and redness of the eyelids. There are nodule with tenderness, slight fever, and headache. The pulse is floating and the tongue is pink with thin and white fur.

Therapeutic Method: Expelling wind and removing heat from the blood

Recipe: Modified *Yinqiao San* (1)
Ingredients:

Flos Lonicerae	30 g
Fructus Forsythiae	15 g
Herba Menthae	9 g
Herba Schizonepetae	9 g
Radix Platycodi	9 g
Fructus Arctii	9 g
Flos Chrysanthemi Indici	12 g
Radix Angelicae Dahuricae	6 g
Radix Paeoniae Rubra	9 g
Radix Scutellariae Praeparata	9 g
Radix Glycyrrhizae	9 g

Administration: Make decoction with the drugs and a proper amount of water and drink the decoction, once a day.

(2) Type of excessive pathogenic heat in the body.

Symptoms and Signs: There are severe swelling, redness and pain of the eyelids. The mass is large or has pustulation. A tumescent lymph node with tenderness is palpable in the preauricular and submaxillary region. There may appear headache, fever, aversion to cold, thirst with preference for drink, dryness of stool, dark brown urine. The pulse is full and rapid and the tongue is red with yellow fur.

Therapeutic Method: Clearing away heat and toxic materials, removing heat from the blood and resolving mass.

Recipe: Modified *Neishu Huanglian Tang* (2)

Ingredients:

Rhizoma Coptidis	9 g
Radix Scutellariae	9 g
Fructus Gardeniae	9 g
Fructus Forsythiae	15 g
Radix et Rhizoma Rhei	6 g
Radix Aucklandiae	6 g
Herba Menthae	9 g
Radix Platycodi	9 g
Radix Paeoniae Rubra	9 g
Radix Scrophulariae	6 g
Radix Trichosanthis	9 g
Radix Angelicae Dahuricae	6 g
Resina Boswelliae Carterii Praeparata	6 g
Radix Glycyrrhizae	12 g

Administration: Make decoction with the drugs and a proper amount of water and drink the decoction. once a day.

2. Other Therapies

(1) Mix *Ruyi Jinhuang San* (84) with some vaseline and apply the mixture to the affected part, twice a day.

(2) Get proper amount of fresh juice from clean Radix Rehemanniae, mix the juice with an equal amount of rice vinegar and apply the mixture to the affected part, four times daily.

(3) Put in a container some common salt and alumen and make solution of them by pouring into the container sufficient

amount of boiling water. Wash the eye with the solution after precipitation.

(4) Blood letting therapy: This therapy requires routine sterilization. Prick with a three-edged needle the homolateral posterior auricular veins to cause bleeding and each time only a vein is pricked for 8-10 drops of blood to be let out. Then prick the acupoint Shaoze with a three-edged needle to cause bleeding.

(5) Acupuncture Therapy: The acupoints commonly chosen are Hegu, Zuanzhu, Tongziliao, Yuyao and Sibai. Two acupoints are punctured at a time, once a day. Retain the needle for ten minutes.

(6) Operation: If the suppuration has been formed, an incision should be made and pus should be removed. Never press the hordeolum.

(7) Propietary: Oral administration of *Lingqiao Jiedu Wan,* 9 g each time, 3 times daily. (101), or *Huanglian Shangqing Wan* (102), 6 g each time, three times daily.

5.2 Lid Abscess

Lid abscess usually develops from the stye. It may also be caused by orbital periostitis, erysipelas of the eyelids or trauma. The disease is termed *Yanyong* in TCM.

Etiology and Pathogenesis

The disease is caused by stagnation of *Qi* and blood following impairment of the *Ying* and Blood systems by pathogenic fire which has flared up to and accumulated in the muscular tissues of the eyelid since its formation as a result of the patient's excessive stomach-fire and preference of pungent and greasy foods. It may also be a result of inward development of a sore which paves the way for invasion of the pathogenic heat into the *Ying* and Blood system and causes accumulation of the evil heat and stagnation of blood, a condition open to necrotic changes. Hence the disease.

Clinical Manifestations

Redness, swelling and burning megalgia of the eyelids, hard and tender eyelids, bulbar conjunctival congestion, edema, or dark blue in color. Tumescent lymph nodes can be palpated in auriculares anteriores and submaxilla.

Type and Treatment

1. Internal Treatment

(1)Type of internal excess of pathogenic fire.

Symptoms and Signs: The symptoms of the eyes are the same as those in 5.1. Other symptoms are headache, pain in the orbit, fever with chills, thirst with preference for drink, poor appetite, dry lips and tongue, dry stool, dark yellow urine, rapid and vigorous pulse and red tongue with yellow fur.

Therapeutic Method: Clearing Away Heat, Purging Fire, Removing Toxic Substances and Promoting Subsidence of Swelling.

Recipe: Modified *Puji Xiaodu Yin* (3)

Ingredients:

Rhizoma Coptidis	9 g
Radix Scutellariae	9 g
Flos Lonicerae	30 g
Fructus Forsythiae	15 g
Radix Isatidis	15 g
Radix Scrophulariae	12 g
Fructus Arctii	12 g
Herba Menthae	9 g

Radix Platycodi	9 g
Radix Bupleuri	6 g
Radix Argelicae Sinensis	12 g
Radix Paeoniae Rubra	9 g
Lignum Sappan	9 g
Radix Glycyrrhizae	9 g

Administration: Decoct the drugs in a proper amount of water and drink the decoction, once a day.

(2) Type of invasion of the body by ulcerous toxin.

Symptoms and Signs: In addition to the symptoms mentioned above, diffused swelling of the face in the periobital areas, high fever with thirsty, and the patient may have flushed face with short breath. The pulse is full and rapid, and the tongue scarlet or dark purplish with thick and yellow fur.

Therapeutic Method: Clearing Up the *Ying* System, Cooling the Blood, Removing Toxic Substances and Promoting Subsidence of Swelling.

Recipe: Modified *Qingying Tang* (4) combined with *Wuwei Xiaodu Yin* (5)

Ingredients:

Radix Rehmanniae	19 g
Cortex Moutan Radicis	9 g
Rhizoma Coptidis	6 g
Fructus Forsythiae	12 g
Flos Lonicerae	30 g
Flos Chrysanthemi Indici	9 g
Herba Taraxaci	15 g
Herba Violae	12 g
Herba Lophatheri	12 g

Semen Plantaginis	12 g
Radix Paeoniae Rubra	9 g
Resina Boswelliae Carterii Praeparata	6 g
Resina Commiphorae Myrrhae Praeparata	6 g
Pulvis Cornu Rhinoceri	1.5 g

In the prescription the drug Pulvis Cornu Rhinoceri is decocted alone or taken temporarily with the hot decoction of the other ingredients, and Semen Plantaginis should be wrapped with gauze and decocted in water with other medicines for oral administration, once a day.

2. Other Therapies

(1) Decoct quantum suffict of Rhizoma Ligustici Chuanxiong, Radix Argelicae Sinensis, Herba Schizonepetae, Spina Gleditsiae and Flos Chrysanthemi Indici in water for fuming and irrigating and hot compressing. Three times daily.

(2) Grind clean Fresh Folium Hibisci into juice and apply it to the affected part. Twice a day.

(3) Propietary: *Niuhuang Jiedu Pian* (103) for oral intake, five tablets a time, three times daily.

(4) Operation: If suppuration has been formed, an incision should be made and the pus removed without pressing.

(5) Antibiotic is used generally.

5.3 Palpebral Erysipelas

The disease is an acute and limited inflammation of the blepharal skin and subcutaneous tissue. It is caused by hemolytic streptococci which usually spread from the face to the eyelids. It is infectious with a sudden onset accompanied by fever, aversion to cold and toxemia. It is termed *Yan Dan* in TCM.

Etiology and Pathogenesis

The disease is due to accumulation of pathogenic heat and stagnation of *Qi* and blood resulting from invasion of the eyelids by exogenous pathogenic wind—heat which accumulates and converts into heat and fire or, it is due to accumulation of dampness—heat in the eyelids as a consequence of upward invasion of wind of the spleen with dampness—heat resulting from retention of pathogenic dampness in the body which stagnates and transforms into heat.

Clinical Manifestations

Burning sensation, swelling and hyperemia of eyelids. The skin in the red swollen region becomes thickened and projecting with small blisters on the affected surface. The margins of the region with pathological changes are clear. In severe cases, local necrosis appears or even spreads around. Apart from a sudden onset, the patient usually has such general symptoms as fever, aversion to cold and headache.

Type and Treatment

1. Internal Treatment

(1) Type of retention of wind—heat.

Symptoms and Signs: The eyelids suffer from red swelling and pain. The part of the affected skin is projected and thickened in pink colour with clear margin. Other symptoms and signs include low fever, aversion to cold, headache, nasal obstruction, general malaise, floating and rapid pulse, pink tongue with thin and white fur.

Therapeutic Method: Expelling Wind and Clearing Away Heat and Pathogenic Factors.

Recipe: Modified *Sanre Xiaodu Yinzi* (6)

Ingredients:

Rhizoma Coptidis	9 g
Radix Scutellariae	9 g
Fructus Forsythiae	15 g
Radix Paeoniae Rubra	9 g
Rhizoma Ligustici Chuanxiong	9 g
Radix Curcumae	9 g
Fructus Arctii	12 g
Herba Menthae	9 g
Radix Angelicae Dahuricae	9 g
Radix Ledebouriellae	9 g
Rhizoma seu Radix Notopterygii	9 g
Radix Glycyrrhizae	12 g

Administration: Decoct the drugs with a proper amount of water and drink the decoction. Once a day.

(2) Type of accumulation of heat and excessiveness of dampness.

Symptoms and Signs: The patient experiences severe pain of the eyelids and has difficulty in opening the eye due to diffuse swelling of the eyelids. The skin is thickened in dark blue colour with a burning feeling, and there are small blisters. Other symptoms and signs include high fever, aversion to cold or thirst with no desire for drink, dark urine, rapid pulse and red tongue with greasy and yellow fur.

Therapeutic Method: Clearing Away Heat and Promoting Diuresis, Subduing Swelling and Alleviating Pain.

Recipe: Modified *Huanglian Jiedu Tang* (7) combined with *San Ren Tang* (8)

Ingredients:

Rhizoma Coptidis	12 g
Radix Scutellariae	9 g
Cortex Phellodendri	6 g
Fructus Gardeniae	12 g
Talcum	30 g
Herba Lophatheri	12 g
Radix Platycodi	12 g
Semen Coicis	15 g
Semen Amomi Cardamomi	9 g
Rhizoma Pinelliae	9 g
Cortex Magroliae Officinalis	9 g
Rhizoma Ligustici Chuanxiong	9 g
Herba Asari	6 g
Rhizoma seu Radix Notoplerygii	9 g

Administration: Decoct the drugs with a proper amount of water and drink the decoction. Once a day.

2. Other Therapies

(1) Decoct Flos Chrysanthemi Indici, Herba Mentha, Herba Schizonepetae and Radix Paeoniae Rubra in water for fumigation and washing, twice a day.

(2) Infuse proper amount of Natrii Sulfas and Calamina with boiling water for hot wet compress, four times daily.

(3) Make a paste with some Indigo Naturalis and sesame oil and apply it to the affected part.

(4) Aricular acupuncture: The commonly used acupoints are eyes, adrenal gland, endocrine and the spleen. Once a day. Retain the needle for 10—15 minutes each time.

5.4 Palpebral Eczema

Palpebral eczema is a disease of palpebral skin characterized by erythema, papular eruption, blister, exudation and formation of scale and scab. If secondary bacterial infection occurs, there will be local suppuration, a condition with pustuliform change. It is usually caused by hypersensitivity to certain allergen or drugs. It is termed *Feng Chi Chuang Yi* in TCM.

Etiology and Pathogenesis

The disease is due to prolonged accumulation of turbid dampness as a result of invasion of the skin by pathogenic dampness which stagnates in the system of superficial resistence, hinders *Qi* of lucid *Yang* from flowing to the skin and causes the turbid dampness in the body not to descend or disperse away. Besides, if the patient has excessive internal damp-ness and heat, they tend to stagnate and thus transform into fire and wind, which will, together with dampness, move upward and accumulate in the eyelid, and cause the disease.

Clinical Manifestations

The patient complains of stabbing itching and burning sensation of the eyelids. The eyelid skin is red and swelling with papule and small blisters which may exudate, ulcerate and scab afterwards. The focus may involve bulbar conjunctiva and cornea, causing congestion and edema of bulbar conjunctiva, superficial infiltration of cornea, etc.

Type and Treatment

1. Internal Treatment

(1) Type of invasion of pathogenic dampness.

Symptoms and Signs: The patient complains of severe itching, slight pain and swelling of the eyelids. Papule and small blisters can be seen on the skin. There are exudation and ulceration. The patient feels tired and listless, and sticky, greasy in the mouth. The pulse is soft and loose, the tongue in pale color with white, slightly thick fur.

Therapeutic Method: Removing Dampness and Toxic Substances, Eliminating the Pathogenic Factors and Relieving Itching.

Recipe: Modified *Chushi Tang* (9)
Ingredient:

Talcum	30 g
Semen Plantaginis	15 g
Caulis Akebiae	6 g
Poria	15 g
Radix Scutellariae	9 g
Radix Coptidis	9 g
Fructus Forsythiae	15 g
Radix Glycyrrhizae	12 g
Rhizoma Atractylodis Praeparata	12 g
Semen Coicis	30 g
Herba Eupatorii	12 g

Administration: Decoct in a proper amount of water the drugs except Semen Plantaginis, which should be wrapped with gauze when decocted. Drink the decoction up as a daily dose: If necessary, the prescription can be used for a few days more though the drugs must be renewed every day.

Modification: for cases with severe itching add:

Radix Angelicae Sinensis	12 g
Radix Paeoniae Rubra	9 g

for cases with severe dampness and erosion add:

Fructus Kochiae	9 g
Radix Sophorae Flavescentis	9 g
Cortex Dictamni Radicis	12 g

(2) Type of stagnation of both dampness and heat.

Symptoms and Signs: Swelling, pain, slight itching and burning sensation of eyelids. There are dermohemia, erosion stink, ropiness and scab, dizziness as if tightly bound, heavy sensation of the body, lassitude, burning sensation of the anus when deficating, scanty deep-colored urine with strangury, smooth and rapid pulse, red tongue with yellow and greasy fur.

Therapeutic Method: Clearing Away Heat, Promoting Diuresis, and Removing Pathogenic Heat from the Blood and Toxic Material from the Body.

Recipe: Modified *Siwu Tang* (10)

Ingredients:

Radix Rehmanniae	12 g
Radix Paeoniae Rubra	9 g
Radix Angelicae Sinensis	9 g
Rhizoma Ligustici Chuanxiong	9 g
Fructus Forsythiae	15 g
Radix Sophorae Flavescentis	15 g
Spica Schizonepetae	9 g
Radix Ledebouriellae	9 g
Herba Menthae Paniculati	9 g
Radix Cynanchi	15 g
Rhizoma Atractylodis Praeparata	12 g
Polyporus Umbellatus	9 g
Flos Lonicerae	15 g

  Cortex Dictamni Radicis   15 g
  Radix Glycyrrhizae   12 g

  Administration: Decoct the drugs in a proper amount of water and drink the decoction for a day's dose. Use the prescription for a few days but the drugs must be renewed every day.

  2. Other Therapies

  (1) Spread the medical powder of *Fulan Xianyan Fang* (85) on the ulcered part.

  (2) Point–injection therapy: The commonly–used acupoints are Dazhui, Feishu, Quchi, Sanyinjiao and Geshu. Each time two of the points are used for injection of 100 mg of vitamin C or vitamin B_1, once a day.

5.5 Chalazion

  Chalazion is a chronic inflammatary granuloma of tarsal glands. It is mostly due to obstruction of the tubes or escapements of the tarsal glands caused by chronic conjunctivitis or blepharitis that results in unsmooth discharge or retention of the glandular excretion. It is termed *Bao Sheng Tan He* in TCM.

Etiology and Pathogenesis

  The cause, production and development of the disease vary. If a patient has dysfunction of the spleen and stomach, improper diet or excessive intake of pungent and / or greasy foods or alcoholic drinks will impair the spleen and stomach. This will lead to debility of the spleen to transport aqueous liquids, and stagnation and accumulation of the liquids will form phlegm. When the phlegm blocks the flow of *Qi* in the channels and lingers too long in the skin and muscles of the eyelid, the disease will occur. If the dampness–phlegm stays in the vessels and channels, the resultant stagnation of *Qi* and blood stasis will produce a mass and cause the disease. Besides, uneliminated stagnation of dampness—phlegm will produce heat when smothering *Yang-Qi*. Once this condition coincides with attacks by exogenous wind and heat, phlegm, dampness and heat will collaborate and further blood stasis. Hence the disease.

Clinical Manifestations

There are heaviness and indisposition in the eyelids. Or the patient may feel as if there were something foreign at the affected part of the eye. The course of the disease progresses slowly. Under the eyelid skin, a round mass of a bean size can be palpated, which is hard, but not red with swelling. When the eye is closed, the eyelid skin projects slightly. There is no adhesion between the skin and the nodule. The corresponding palpebral conjunctiva shows a regional purlish red color.

Type and Treatment

1. Internal Treatment

(1) Type of stagnation of phlegm—dampness.

Symptoms and Signs: The patient complains of foreign body sensation or heaviness and discomfort of the affected eye. The eyelid skin projects. A nodule is palpated without pain. There are lassitude and weakness, poor appetite sticky and greasy mouth, thready and soft pulse, thick and pale tongue with white and greasy fur.

Therapeutic Method: Removing dampness and resolving phlegm, promoting blood circulation and dissolving mass.

Recipe: Modified *Huajian Erchen Wan* (11)

Ingredients:

Rhizoma Pinelliae Praeparata	9 g
Pericarpium Citri Reticulatae	9 g

Poria	12 g
Rhizoma Coptidis	9 g
Thallus Laminariae seu Eckloniae	12 g
Bombyx Batryticatus	6 g
Bulbus Fritillariae Thunbergii	12 g
Radix Angelicae Dahuricae	9 g
Radix Curcumae	9 g
Squama Manitis	9 g

Administration: Decoct the drugs in a proper amount of water and drink the decoction, once a day.

(2) Type of accumulation of heat due to phlegm-dampness.

Symptoms and Signs: The patient complains of foreign body sensation in the affected eye with local eminence, and slight pain when the nodule is palpated. The corresponding palpebral conjunctival is congestive in purplish red color. The pulse is soft and a little rapid and the tongue is red with greasy fur.

Therapeutic Method: Clearing away heat and promoting diuresis, resolving the hard lump

Recipe: Modified *Fangfeng Sanjie Tang* (12)

Ingredients:

Radix Ledebouriellae	9 g
Radix Angelicae Pubescentis	6 g
Flos Carthami	9 g
Lignum Sappan	12 g
Radix Angelicae Sinensis	9 g
Pollen Typhae	9 g
Talcum	30 g
Excrementum Bombycis	12 g
Flos Lonicerae	30 g

Rhizoma Smilacis Glabrae	15 g
Fructus Forsythiae	12 g
Radix Glycyrrhizae	12 g
Retinervus Luffae Fructus	15 g

Administration: Decoct the drugs in a proper amount of water and drink the decoction, once a day.

2. Other Therapics

(1) Decoct equal quantities of Flos Chrysanthemi Indici, Spina Gleditsiae, Flos Carthami and Lignum Sappan in water for hot compress, three times daily.

(2) Mix *Zijin Ding* (86) with water and apply the mixture to the affected skin. twice a day.

(3) Operation: If the nodule is too large and is not absorbed for a considerable period, incision and curettage should be made.

5.6 Blepharitis Cilistis

The disease is a subacute or chronic inflammation of the margin of the lid surface, eyelash hair follicle and the gland body tissues. It is usually caused by bacterial infection and the most common are staphylococci and Morax—axenfeld diplococci. In addition, it may also be induced by conjunctiva inflammation and chemical and physical irritation. It is termed *Jian Xuan Chi Lan* in TCM.

Etiology and Pathogenesis

The disease is caused by long standing retention of dampness—heat in the eyelids as a consequence of accumulation of dampness—heat in the spleen due to excessive intake of pungent and greasy foods, Apart from this, when exogenous pathogenic wind and heat attack the skin and stay in the eyelid, they will cause obstruction of the sweat pores: a condition that will lead to dysfunction of the defending *Qi* in combatting diseases, and to malnutrition of the eyelid skin. The disease will then occur.

Clinical Manifestations

The patient complains of photophobia and lacrimation or a sensation of irritative itching in the margin of the lid. There are branny desquamations attached at the eyelash-roots, or small pustulae growing on the margins of the lid. The herpes may rupture and scab. Under the crusts are ulcers. There are hyperemia of the lid margins, pachynsis and deplumation. The eyelashes will not renewable on account of destruction of follicles. In some cases hyperemia and erosion may appear in the two canthus, usually accompanied with a sensation of urtication.

Type and Treatment

1. Internal Treatment

(1) Type of hyperactivity of pathogenic dampness-heat.

Symptoms and Signs: The patient experiences photophobia and lacrimation, constant stabbing pain or itching sensation. There are red erosion, ropiness and bleeding ulcers, exudation and ulceration on the margins of the lids. Other symptoms include dry and greasy mouth, thirsty with no desire to drink, rapid pulse, red tongue with greasy and quite light yellow fur.

Therapeutic Method: Clearing away heat, drying dampness, dispelling wind and arresting itching

Recipe: Modified *Zaoshi Tang* (13)

Ingredients:

Rhizoma Coptidis	9 g
Fructus Gardeniae	9 g

Rhizoma Atractylodis	9 g
Rhizoma Atractylodis Macrocephalae	12 g
Rhizoma Dioscoreae	15 g
Pericarpium Citri Reticulatae	9 g
Rhizoma Pinlliae	9 g
Fructus Aurantii	12 g
Rhizoma Picrorhizae	6 g
Cortex Fraxini	9 g
Radix Ledebouriellae	9 g
Cortex Dictamni Radicis	12 g
Fructus Kochiae	12 g
Radix Glycyrrhizae	9 g

Administration: Decoct the drugs in a proper amount of water and drink the decoction, once a day.

(2) Type of invasion of pathogenic wind-heat.

Symptoms and Signs: There are light redness in the lid margins, peculiar itching and photophobia. Attachment of the branny scales are seen at the bases of the lashes. There are hyperemia of the lid margins, headache with aversion to wind, dry throat with pain, floating rapid pulse and red tongue with thin yellow fur.

Therapeutic Method: Expelling wind to relieve itching and removing pathogenic heat from blood

Recipe: Modified *Chaihu San* (14)

Ingredients:

Radix Bupleuri	15 g
Herba Schizonepetae	9 g
Radix Ledebouriellae	12 g
Rhizoma seu Radix	9 g

Radix Paeoniae Rubra	9 g
Radix Rehmanniae	9 g
Radix Platycodi	9 g
Rhizoma Cimicifugae	6 g
Cortex Dictamni Radicis	12 g
Flos Lonicerae	15 g
Herba Taraxaci	15 g
Herba Menthae	9 g
Folium Nelumbinis	9 g
Radix Glycyrrhizae	9 g

Administration: Decoct the drugs in a proper amount of water and drink the decoction, once a day.

(3) Type of deficiency of the spleen with internal dampness.

Symptoms and Signs: The patient complains of slight itching and pain on the margin of the lid. There are redness of the lid margin, mostly with eczematoid blisters, ulcer and ropiness or exudation and erosion. Other symptoms include poor appetite, lassitude, a pale and thick tongue with white thick fur and soft, weak pulse.

Therapeutic Method: Invigorating the Spleen and Eliminating Dampness Recipe: Modified *Huangqi Tang* (15)

Ingredients:

Radix Astragali sue Hedysar	30 g
Poria	15 g
Rhizoma Dioscoreae Praeparata	15 g
Rhizoma Atractylodis Macrocephalae Praeparata	12 g
Rhizoma Cimicifugae	6 g
Fructus Aurantii praeparata	9 g
Pericărpium Citri Reticulatae	6 g

Radix Ledebouriellae	9 g
Rhizoma seu Radix Notopterygii	9 g
Zaocys	6 g
Herba Agastachis	12 g
Herba Spirodelae	9 g
Radix Glycyrrhizae	12 g

Administration: Decoct the drugs in a proper amount of water and drink the decoction, once a day.

2. Other therapies

(1) Decoct Herba Senecionis Scandentis, Flos Chrysanthemi Indici Herba Taraxaci, Herba Schizonepetae, Radix Ledebouriellae and Old Tea in water for fuming and irrigating, three times daily.

(2) Decoct Flos Chrysanthemi Indici and Alumen in water and wash the eyes with the decoction after its clarification, three times daily.

(3) Phoenix oil: Boil an egg and remove the egg-white. put the yolk in a spoon, cook it with mild fire and stir it continuously until it changes into an oil. Dip a glass stick into the oil and apply the oil on the stick to the affected part.

(4) Bake Excrementa Bombycum and grind it into powder. Mix the powder with sesame oil or vinegar to form a paste. Apply the paste to the affected part.

5.7 Ptosis (Blepharoptosis)

The disease means there are difficulties in raising the upper eyelid that affect vision because the dropping eyelid covers the pupil partly or completely. The disease is classified into two types: congenital and acquired. The acquired type will be dealt with in this chapter. It is usually due to injury to the levator muscle of the upper eyelid or oculomotor nerve or due to myasthenia gravis of unknown etiology. It is termed *Shang Bao Xia Chui* in TCM.

Etiology and Pathogensis

When a person has deficiency of spleen–*Qi*, he / she will suffer from malnutrition of the eyelid due to sinking of *Qi* of Middle–*Jiao*, a condition meaning dysfunction of the spleen in transporting refined nutrient substances to the eyelid. Then, as the eyelid cannot get nourished as usual, it will become too weak to raise itself. Besides, if one gets tired with much sweating, the superficial texture and the pores will be open and exogenous pathogenic wind will take this advantage to invade into and stay in the eyelid, interfering with normal flow of *Qi* and blood in the channels and vessels and causing stagnation of *Qi* and blood stasis that hinder supply of nutrient to the eyelid skin, and the disease will occur.

Clinical Manifestations

The eyelid is loosely dropping and the patient finds it difficult to raise the eyelid. The disease may affect one eye or both of the eyes. In mild cases, the pupil is half covered. In severe cases, the upper eyelid entirely loses its ability to raise itself and covers the whole cornea. The patient usually takes a characteristic posture with the head thrown back in seeing things.

Type and Treatment

1. Internal Treatment

(1) Type of insufficiency of the spleen–*Qi*.

Symptoms and Signs: Usually both the upper eyelids are dropping. The dropping is mild in the morning but gradually becomes severe. It becomes mild after resting but worse after working. In some cases, the disease may be accompanied by disturbance in eye movement. Other symptoms include lassitude, general weakness, pale and thick tongue with toothprint, thin and yellow fur, small and weak pulse.

Therapeutic Method: Strengthening the spleen and invigorating vital function, nourishing the spleen and replenishing *Qi*

Recipe: Modified *Buzhong Yiqi Tang* (16)

Ingredients:

Radix Astragali seu Hedysari	30 g
Radix Codonopsis Pilosulae	15 g
Radix Glycyrrhizae Praeparata	12 g
Rhizoma Atractylodis Macrocephalae	15 g
Pericarpium Citri Reticulatae	9 g
Rhizoma Cimicifugae	6 g
Radix Puerariae	9 g
Radix Bupleuri	12 g
Radix Argelicae Sinensis	15 g
Radix Paeoniae Alba	30 g

Administration: Decoct the drugs in a proper amount of water and drink the decoction, once a day.

Modification: For cases with deficiency of blood, add:

Caulis Spatholobi	30 g
Radix Polygoni Multiflori	15 g

For cases with severe ptosis, add:

Rhizoma Ligustici Chuanxiong	6 g
Retinervus Luffae Fructus	15 g
Radix Saviae Miltiorrhizae	30 g
Radix Ginseng	15 g

For cases with loose stools, add:

| Rhizoma Zingiberis Praeparata | 6 g |
| Radix Aconiti Praeparata | 6 g |

For cases with lassitude, sticky and greasy mouth, add:

Herba Eupatorii	15 g
Rhizoma Atractylidis Praeparata	12 g
Fructus Amomi	9 g

(2) Type of invasion of channels and vessels by pathogenic wind.

Symptoms and Signs: Sudden onset and obvious dropping of upper eyelid, which usually affects one eye. There is hypoesthesia or anesthesia in the eyelid skin, with disturbance in eye movement, headache, and feeling of fullness in the head. The tongue is pink with thin white fur and the pulse floating and unsmooth.

Therapeutic Method: Expelling wind, regulating blood flow and removing obstruction in the channels

Recipe: Modified *Zhuyang Hexue Tang* (17)

Ingredients:

Radix Astragali seu Hedysari	30 g
Rhizoma Cimicifugae	9 g
Radix Glycyrrhizae Praeparata	9 g
Radix Angelicae Sinensis	12 g
Radix Paeoniae Alba	30 g
Radix Bupleuri	15 g
Radix Ledebouriellae	12 g
Radix Puerariae	15 g
Ramulus Uncariae cum Uncis	12 g
Radix Angelicae Dahuricae	9 g
Rhizoma seu Radix Notopterygii	9 g

Administration: Decoct the drugs in a proper amount of water and drink the decoction, once a day.

Put Ramulus Uncarial cum Uncis into the pot after the water and the medicines have been boiled for five minutes.

Modification: For cases with ecchymosis on the surface of the longue, add:

Radix Salviae Miltiorrhizae	30 g
Radix Curcumae	12 g
Caulis Spatholobi	30 g
Rhizoma Ligustici Chuanxiong	6 g

For cases with fever and aversion to cold, add:

Flos Lonicerae	30 g
Fructus Forsythiae	15 g
Herba Menthae	9 g

2. Other Therapies

(1) Bake Rhizoma Zingiberis Recens slices for hot compress to the eyelid skin, three times daily.

(2) Acupuncture: The commonly used acupoints are Zanzhu, Sizhu Kong, Yuyao, Zusanli, Pishuand, Hegu. Each time use two periocular points and two distal points, once a day.

(3) Moxibustion: Moxibustion is applied to Sanyinjiao, twenty minutes each time, once a day.

(4) Propietary: *Renshen Jianpi Wan* (104) for oral administration, 9 g. a time, three times daily.

6 Diseases of the Lacrimal Apparatus

Diseases of the lacrimal apparatus belong to the category of diseases of the canthus in TCM. Canthus correspond to the heart, representing *Qi* oriculus in the five oriculi. Therefore diseases of the canthus have a close relation with the heart. The heart dominates fire and governs blood circulation. Fire flaring up due to exuberance of the heart *Qi*, will result in accumulation and upward reversed flow of *Qi* and blood and obstruct the vessels and channels, when the fire gets stagnant in the canthus, the diseases occur. Both canthus are exposed to the outside and apt to be attacked by wind, heat and fire pathogens. The combined accumulation of them in the canthus may also cause disease. Tears are generated by the liver, so epiphora is usually related to insufficiency of the liver blood, and to deficiency of the liver and kidney. In treating the diseases of both canthi, methods of clearing away heat and expelling pathogenic factors, removing the heart fire, warming and recuperating the liver and kidney are commonly used.

6.1 Dysfunction of the Lacrimal Apparatus

Dysfunction of the lacrimal apparatus refers to epiphora without any organic pathologic change of the lacrimal passage. When the lacrimal passage is douched, the fluid passes freely, but when a colored fluid is dropped into the conjunctiva sac, no such fluid flows out from the nasal cavity. Epiphora is caused by inadequate drainage or retention of tears. It is termed *Leng Lei Zheng* in TCM.

Etiology and Pathogenesis

This syndrome is often caused by deficiency of the liver and kidney. There are fluids in five *Zang*—organs and six *Fu*—organs. The fluid of the liver flowing to the eyes is called tears, and controlled by the liver. Therefore, the liver has a close relationship with tears. The liver and kidney have a common source. When the liver and kidney fail to control their fluids due to deficiency, tears overflow and the disease occurs. In addition, endopathic wind resulting from deficiency of blood or exogenous pathogenic wind attacking the eye may cause dysfunction of the lacrimal apparature and lead to the disease.

Clinical Manifestations

Epiphora which may become worse when the eye is exposed to wind, but with no photophobia. There are blepharochalasis, weakened orbicular muscles of the eye, hypotension of the lacrimal sac, loose contact of the lacrimal punctum with the eyeball, free lacrimal passage or with little resistance when irrigated.

Type and Treatment

1. Internal Treatment

(1) Type of deficiency of the liver and kidney.

Symptoms and Signs: dryness of the eye, blurred vision, dizziness, lassitude in the loins and knees, deep and thready pulse, red and uncoated tongue.

Therapeutic Method: Warming and tonifying the liver and kidney, arresting of secretion and controlling tears.

Recipe: Modified *Shenqi Wan* (18)
Ingredients:

Rhizoma Rehmanniae Praeparatae	9 g
Fructus Corni	9 g
Fructus Ligustri Lucidi	15 g
Rhizoma Dioscoreae	9 g
Poria	12 g
Cortex Cinnamomi	6 g
Radix Aconiti Praeparata	6 g
Herba Cistanchis	12 g
Semen Cuscutae	15 g
Fructus Schisandrae	9 g
Radix Ophiopogonis	12 g
Radix Paeoniae Alba	15 g
Radix Glycyrrhizae	9 g

Administration: Decoct the above drugs in water for oral dose. One dose daily.

(2) Type of attack of wind due to blood deficiency.

Symptoms and Signs: Usually there are dryness and itching in both eyes, frequent lacrimation, epiphora worsened by exposure to wind with thin, clear lacrimal secretion, dry mouth and lips, dim complexion, deep and weak pulse, reddened tip of the tongue, and little coating.

Therapeutic Method: Nourishing the blood and promoting production of the body fluid, expelling wind and arresting tears.

Recipe: Modified *Zhilei Bugan San* (19)
Ingredients:

Radix Angelicae Sinensis	15 g
Radix Paeoniae Alba	18 g

Rhizoma Rehmanniae Praeparatae	9 g
Rhizoma Ligustici Chuanxiong	6 g
Fructus Tribuli Alba	9 g
Radix Ledebouriellae	9 g
Radix Glycyrrhizae	9 g
Cortex Dictamni Radicis	9 g

Administration: Decoct the above drugs in water for oral dose, once a day.

Modification: For cases with weakness and lassitude, add:

Radix Astragali seu Hedysari	15 g
Radix Codonopsis Pilosulae	12 g

For cases with copious tears in winter, intolerance of cold, and cold limbs, add:

Herba Asari	6 g
Ramulus Cinnamoni	12 g

2. Other Therapies

(1) Make a mixture with equal amount of crucian carp bile and human milk, and instil a bit of the mixture into the eyes, 3 times a day.

(2) Acupuncture: The commonly relected acupoints are Jingming, Qiuhou, Chengqi, Yangbai, Ganshu, Shenshu, and Hegu. Needle 4 points each time, once a day. Retain the needles for 20 minutes. When needling Jingming, insert the needle on to the nasal bone, using peck manipulation. At the moment when the patien gets needling sensations the needle may be withdrawn a little immediately then retain the needle for 20 minutes.

(3) Propietary: *Qiju Dihuang Wan* (110) or *Shiquan Dabu Wan* (105) for oral administration: 1 bolus each time, 3 times a day.

6.2 Chronic Dacryocystitis

Chronic dacryocystitis is characterized by mucous purulent secretion flowing from the puncta when pressure is applied to the sac. As the nasolacrimal duct is obstructed, tears may accumulate in the lacrimal sac for a long time, leading to congestion and thickening of the sac lining and reproduction of bacteria in the sac. It is termed *Loujing* in TCM.

Etiology and Pathogenesis

The disease is due to attack of summer heat and dampness to the puncta lacrimalis, or due to dampness-heat in the spleen that moves along the Urinary Bladder Channel of Foot-Taiyang, accumulates in the inner canthus and results in suppuration. Besides, when the patient happens to be in a state of deficiency of *Qi* and blood, exogenous pathogenic wind-heat may invade into the puncta lacrimalis. and the patient's resistence will be too weak to expel the pathogens out, leading to accumulation of the pathogens and giving rise to suppuration. Hence the disease.

Clinical Manifestations

Epiphora, with pus discharge at times. The color and lustre of the skin of the region of lacrimal sac is normal. By pressing upon the sac, mucous or purulent secretion escapes from puncta. In some cases, an undulatory cystis is palpable in the region of the lacrimal sac. When the lacrimal sac is irrigated, the fluid can not pass through the passage.

Type and Treatment

1. Internal Treatment

(1) Type of retention of dampness-heat in the interior.

Symptoms and Signs: Usually the patient may feel distension

and discomfort in the region of the inner canthi. There are epiphora, viscid lacrimal secretion. Profuse tears accumulate in the palpebral tissue. By pressing the region of lacrimal sac, large amount of tears and purluent secretion may flow out. The patient may feel heaviness in the head, depressed feeling in the chest, thirst but having no desire for drinking, slippery and slightly rapid pulse, reddened tongue, and greasy yellowish fur.

Therapeutic Method: Clearing away heat and promoting diuresis, promoting blood circulation and discharging pus

Recipe: Modefied *Xiepi Chure Yin* (20)

Ingredients:

Rhizoma Coptidis	9 g
Radix Scutellariae	9 g
Radix et Rhizoma Rhei	3 g
Natrii Sulfas	6 g
Radix Astragali seu Hedysari	15 g
Radix Angelicae Dahuricae	6 g
Radina Boswelliae Carterii Praeparata	9 g
Radix Platycodi	9 g
Herba Lophatheri	12 g
Flos Lonicerae	30 g
Fructus Forsythiae	15 g
Radix Glycyrrhizae	12 g

Administration: Decoct the above drugs in water for oral dose, one dose daily.

(2) Type of weakened body resistance and lingering pathogenic factors.

Symptoms and Signs: There are epiphora, watery or viscid lacrimal secretion, but the skin of the region of lacrimal sac is in normal color. By pressing upon the region of lacrimal sac, watery or thin purluent secretion will flow out and the course may last long. Other symptoms and signs include weakness and lassitude, loose stools, thready and weak pulse, pale tongue, with thin and white fur.

Therapeutic Method: Strengthening the body resistance and eliminating pus, clearing away heat to expel pathogenic factors

Recipe: Modified *Qianjin Tuoli San* (21)

Ingredients:

Radix Astragali seu Hedysari	24 g
Radix Codonopsis Pilosulae	12 g
Poria	12 g
Radix Puerariae	12 g
Radix Paeoniae Alba	15 g
Radix Angelicae Sinensis	9 g
Rhizoma Ligustici Chuanxiong	9 g
Radix Platycodi	9 g
Spina Gleditsiae	6 g
Radix Glycyrrhizae	9 g

Administration: Decoct the above drugs in water for oral dose, one dose daily.

2. Other therapies

Surgical Treatment: Dacryocystorhinostomy or dacryocystectomy are prescribed for patients who fail to respond positively to the therapy.

6.3 Acute Dacryocystitis

Acute Dacryocystitis is an acute suppurative inflammation of the lacrimal sac. It may develop from the secondary infection in the course of chronic decryocystitis or occur acutely without any obstruction of lacrimal passage. It is termed *Loujing Chuang* in TCM.

Etiology and pathogenesis

The disease is caused by pathogenic wind—heat which goes up along the channels of Taiyang and accumulates in the inner canthi after it has invaded into the body. The disease may also be due to accumulation of excessive heat in the Heart Channel that attacks the vessels and inner canthi, and results in slough there.

Clinical Manifestations

The patient suffers from severe pain and has a burning sensation in the region of the lacrimal sac. The pain may radiate to the frontal part. These symptoms are often accompanied by headache, fever, aversion to cold, general malaise, heavy red swelling in the region of the sac and the surrounding skin, a hard mass which could be touched on the region of the sac, exquisite tenderness, submaxillary and preauricular lymphadenectasis.

Type and Treatment

1. Internal Treatment

(1) Type of excessive wind—heat.

Symptoms and Signs: Lacrimation with pain, congestion and swelling of the skin over the sac, tenderness, a palpable nodule in the region of the sac, aversion to wind, fever, floating, rapid pulse, reddened tongue with thin yellow fur.

Therapeutic Method: Dispelling wind, purging intense heat, and removing heat from the blood.

Recipe: Modified *Zhuye Xiejing Tang* (22)

Ingredients:

Herba Lophatheri   12 g

Rhizoma Coptidis	9 g
Radix et Rhizoma Rhei	3 g
Fructus Gardeniae	9 g
Radix Scutellariae	9 g
Rhizoma Alismatis	9 g
Poria	12 g
Radix Bupleuri	9 g
Radix Angelicae Dahuricae	9 g
Radix Ledebouriellae	9 g
Radix Platycodi	9 g
Flos Lonicerae	30 g
Fructus Forsythiae	15 g
Herba Taraxaci	30 g

Administration: Decoct the above drugs in water for oral dose. One dose daily.

(2) Type of excessive noxious—heat.

Symptoms and Signs: Severe pain in the region of the sac with a burning sensation, localized congestion, dark blue swelling of the skin extending arround, a palpable tender mass, lymphadenectasis which could be felt in the submaxillary and preauricular region, fever, aversion to cold, dry mouth, thirst, full and forceful pulse, reddened tongue with yellow fur.

Therapeutic Method: Clearing away toxic material, purging intense heat and dissolving swelling.

Recipe: Modified *Nei Shu Huanglian* Tang (2)

Ingredients:

Rhizoma Coptidis	9 g
Radix Scutellariae	9 g
Fructus Gardeniae	9 g

Fructus Forsythiae	12 g
Herba Menthae	9 g
Radix Platycodi	9 g
Radix et Ehizoma Rhei	3 g
Radix Angelicae Dahuricae	9 g
Resina Commiphorae Myrrhae Praeparata	6 g
Lignum Sappan	9 g
Flos Chrysanthemi Indici	12 g
Radix Achyranthis Bidentatae	9 g
Radix Scrophulariae	9 g
Radix Glycyrrhizae	9 g

Administration: Decoct the above drugs in water for oral dose. One dose daily.

2. Other Therapies:

(1) If suppuration has not yet taken form, apply *"Zi Jin Ding"* (86) to the affected site twice a day.

(2) Pound fresh Folium Chrysanthemi Indici (15 g.), and brown sugar (just the right amount) in a mortar, apply the paste to the affected part, twice a day.

(3) Flos Lonicerae	30 g
Flos Chrysanthemi Indici	15 g
Lignum Sappan	9 g

Administration: Decoct the drugs in water for hot compress, 3 times a day.

(4) Surgical Treatment: If suppuration occurs, an incision should be made for pus-discharge. If there is fistula, the sac should be extirpated after inflammation is controlled.

(5) Propietary: *Niuhuang Qingxin Wan* (106) for oral administration, 9 g, a time, three times daily.

7 Diseases of the Conjunctiva

The conjunctiva is located at the anteria surface of the eyeball and so it is susceptible to diseases caused by exogenous pathogenic factors. The bulbar conjunctiva is the white part of the eye. In TCM, it is termed *Baijing*. The palpebral conjunctiva is considered a component part of the eyelid. In terms of the Five Orbiculi, *Baijing* (the bulbar conjunctiva) corresponds to the lung and falls into *Qi* Orbiculus. The eyelid corresponds to the spleen and falls into Flesh Orbiculus. Therefore, diseases of the conjunctiva have close relationship with the lung and spleen, and are usually caused by obstruction of the lung *Qi*, deficiency of the lung— *Yin* or dampness—heat in the spleen channel. In treatment, such therapies as dispelling wind and removing heat, promoting the flow of lung—*Qi*, nourishing *Yin* to moisten the lung and expelling damp—heat are often used.

7.1 Trachoma

Trachoma is a chronic infective conjunctivitis caused by trachoma chlamydia. Occasionally, the disease may begin acutely and then become a chronic inflammation. At the late stage, many complications may occur and even result in blindness. It is termed *Jiao Chuang* in TCM.

Etiology and Pathogenesis

When retention of endogenouse dameness and heat is worsened by exogenous pathogenic wind and heat, there will appear obstruction by dampness and heat. Moreover, they will join the intruding pathogenic wind and heat in attacking the eye, resulting in blockage of the vessels of the eyelid and stagnation of *Qi* and blood stasis there. Then the disease occurs, the blockage of the eyelid vessels may also be caused by excessive heat in the blood which is transferred from middle *Jiao* with hyperactive heat. This will lead to the disease.

Clinical Manifestations

In mild cases, there may be no subjective symptoms or there is just a foreign body sensation, epiphora induced by wind, profuse eye secretion. In severe cases or cases with complication, there may be photophobia, lacrimation, sticky eye secretion, asthenopia, and some other symptoms such as swelling and congestion of the upper palpebral conjunctiva and the fornices, blurred vessels, rough conjunctival surface, hypertrophic papilla, felliculosis. At the early stage, examinations may reval pannus and grayish-white superficial infiltration on the upper corneal limbus, hypertrophy of the conjunctiva with gray-white networklike scars in varying size. At the late stage, there may be such complications as ptosis of the upper eyelid, entropion, trichiasis, corneal ulcer, corneal pannus, symblepharom xerosis, dacryocystitis, etc.

Type and Treatment

1. Internal Treatment

(1) Type of retention of endogenous dampness and heat.

Symptoms and Signs: Ophthalmalgia with dry, photophobia, lacrimation, sticky eye secretion, slightly swollen eyelid, papillary hypertrophy of the palpebral conjunctiva, large amount of the conjunctival follicles, slight congestion of the bulbar conjunctiva, corneal pannus, lassitude, anorexia, sticky mouth, rapid and slippery pulse, reddened tongue, yellow and sticky coating.

Therapeutic Method: Clearing away heat, eliminating dampness, removing heat from the blood and dissipating blood stasis.

Recipe: Modified *Chufeng Qingpi Yin* (23)
Ingredients:

Spica Schizonepetae	9 g
Radix Platycodi	12 g
Radix Ledebouriellae	9 g
Rhizoma Coptidis	9 g
Fructus Forsythiae	15 g
Rhizoma Anemarrhenae	6 g
Natrii Sulfas Exsiccatus	6 g
Radix et Rhizoma Rhei	3 g
Pericarpium Citri Reticulatae	9 g
Gypsum Fibrosum	30 g
Radix Rehmanniae	9 g
Cortex Fraxini	9 g
Radix Glycyrrhizae	12 g

Administration: Decoct the above drugs in water for oral dose. One dose daily.

Modification: for cases with sevsre itching, add:

Fructus Tribuli	12 g
Cortex Dictamni Radicis	9 g
Radix Sophorae Flavescentis	9 g

for cases with marked congestion in the eyelids add:

Lignum Sappan	9 g
Cortex Moutan Radicis	9 g
Radix Paeoniae Rubra	9 g

(2) Type of excessiveness of wind and heat.

Symptoms and Signs: Dryness and discomfort of the eyes, foreign body sensation, itching with slight pain, lacrimation induced by wind, small papilla with a few follicles on the bulbar conjunctiva, dry mouth and pharyngodynia, floating and rapid pulse, reddish tongue with thin and yellow coating.

Therapeutic Method: Dispelling wind, removing heat, eliminating pathogenic heat from the blood and alleviating itching.

Recipe: Modified *Qingpi Liangxie Tang* (24)

Ingredients:

Radix Ledebouriellae	12 g
Herba Schizonepetae	9 g
Cortex Dictamni Radicis	9 g
Periostracum Cicadae	9 g
Flos Chrysanthemi	9 g
Fructus Kochiae	9 g
Pericarpium Citri Reticulatae	9 g
Rhizoma Atractylodis	9 g
Cortex Magnoliae Officinalis	6 g
Fructus Forsythiae	15 g
Radix Paeoniae Rubra	9 g
Radix et Rhizoma Rhei	3 g
Cortex Moutan Radicis	9 g
Radix Glycyrrhizae	9 g

Administration: Decoct the above drugs in water for oral dose. Once a day.

(3) Type of excessiveness of pathogenic heat in the interior.

Symptoms and Signs: Photophobia, lacrimation, severe stabbiong pain, profuse eye secretion, palpebral conjunctival congestion, diffuse papillary hypertrophy, folliculosis, bulbar conjunctival congestion, corneal pannus, constipation, dark yellow urine, thirst for drink, rapid and large pulse, reddened tongue with yellow coating.

Therapeutic Method: Clearing away heat, purging pathogenic fire, removing heat from the blood and dissipating blood stasis.

Recipe: Modified *Guishao Honghua San* (25)
Ingredients:

Radix Angelicae Sinensis	12 g
Radix Paeoniae Rubra	9 g
Flos Carthami	9 g
Radix et Rhizoma Rhei	3 g
Radix Rehmanniae	9 g
Radix Scutellariae	9 g
Fructus Gardeniae	9 g
Fructus Forsythiae	12 g
Radix Isatidis	15 g
Radix Cynanchi Paniculati	15 g
Radix Ledebouriellae	9 g
Radix Angelicae Dahuricae	9 g
Radix Glycyrrhizae	9 g

Administration: Decoct the above drugs in water for oral dose. Once a day.

2. Other Therapies

(1) Eye droppings of *Waizhang Yanyaoshui* (87) four times a day.

(2) Eye droppings of *Huanglian Xiguashuang Yanyaoshui* (80) four times a day.

(3) Decoct equal amounts of Cortex Mori Radicis, Dried Alum and Salt in water, precipitate the decoction and use the precipitated decoction as an eye lotion to wash the eyes.

(4) Acupuncture treatment: Needle the points of Zusanli, Xuehai, Taichong with strong stimulation once a day.

7.2 Acute Catarrhal Conjunctivitis

The disease is characterized by marked congestion of the bulbar conjunctiva with muco-purulent discharge. Usually it is caused by staphylococci, pneumococci, streptococci and Koch-weeks bacilli, through direct contact infection. It is termed *Baofeng Kere* in TCM.

Etiology and Pathogenesis

If exogenous pathogenic wind and heat has invaded into the body through the integument and musculature, they tend to attack upper *Jiao*, firstly the lung, resulting in wind and heat in the lung channel. When the resultant wind and heat flare up to the eye, the disease occurs. Besides, if a person with constant excessive endogenous heat due to hyperactive *Yang* is attacked by pathogenic exogenous wind and heat, the original endogenous heat may combine with the intensive pathogens, flare up to the eye and cause the disease.

Clinical Manifestations

The patient may have a foreign body sensation, or even a burning pain in severe cases, with photophobia, lacrimation and profuse eye secretion which may even seal the palpebral tissure in the morning. The other symptoms includide palpebral conjunctival congestion, even swelling eyelid, bulbar conjunctival congestion or edema, petechial or patchy subconjunctival hemorrhage which can be seen in severe cases.

Type and Treatment

1. Internal Treatment

(1) Type of overactivity of pathogenic wind—heat.

Symptoms and Signs: These include itching and discomfort, foreign body sensation, photophobia and lacrimation, comparatively scanty and thin secretion, slightly red swollen eyelid, bulbar conjunctival congestion, headache, stuffy nose, aversion to wind, slight fever, floating and rapid pulse, pink tongue with thin, white coating.

Therapeutic Method: Promoting dispersing function of the lung, dispelling wind, clearing away heat and cooling the blood.

Recipe: Modified *Qufeng Sanre Yinzi* (26)

Ingredients:

Fructus Arctii	12 g
Rhizoma seu Radix Notopterygii	9 g
Radix Ledebouriellae	9 g
Herba Menthae	9 g
Flos Chrysanthemi	9 g
Folium Mori	9 g
Frucrus Forsythiae	12 g
Fructus Gardeniae	9 g
Radix et Rhizoma Rhei	3 g
Radix Paeoniae Rubra	9 g
Radix Angelicae Sinensis	9 g
Rhizoma Ligustici Chuanxiong	6 g

Administration: Decoct them above drugs in water for oral dose. Once a day.

(2) Type of overactivity of lung—heat.

Symptoms and Signs: Photophobia and lacrimation, burning pain, profuse sticky secretion, palpebral edema, bulbar conjunctival edema and congestion in brilliant red color, thirst, dry throat and cough, dry stools, rapid pulse, reddened tongue with thin, yellowish coating.

Therapeutic Method: Clearing away heat, purging pathogenic fire, dispelling pathogenic wind.

Recipe: Modified *Xiefei Yin* (27)

Ingredients:

Gypsum Fibrosum	30 g
Radix Scutellariae	12 g
Cortex Mori Radicis	9 g
Radix Ophiopogonis	9 g
Fructus Gardeniae	9 g
Fructus Forsythiae	15 g
Poria Rubra	9 g
Caulis Akebiae	9 g
Rhizoma seu Radix Notopterygii	9 g
Herba Spirodelae	12 g
Flos Chrysanthemi	9 g
Cortex Moutan Radicis	9 g
Radix Paeoniae Rubra	12 g
Radix Glycyrrhizae	9 g

Administration: Decoct the above drugs in water for oral dose. One dose daily.

(3) Type of excessiveness of pathogenic fire in the liver and lung.

Symptoms and Signs: The symptoms are the same as the last type. In addition, spotted grayish-white opacities can be found in the superficial layers of the cornea. There is hypochondriac pain, bitter taste in the mouth, dryness of throat rapid and taut pulse, reddened margin of the tongue with thin, yellowish coating.

Therapeutic Method: Purging the liver of its pathogenic fire, promoting dispersing function of the lung, and removing heat from the blood.

Recipe: Modified *Qinggan San* (28)

Ingredients:

Radix Scatellariae	9 g
Radix Gentianae	9 g
Radix Bupleuri	9 g
Cortex Moutan Radicis	9 g
Cortex Mori Radicis	9 g
Cortex Lycii Radicis	9 g
Radix Rehmanniae	9 g
Radix et Rhizoma Rhei	6 g
Herba Menthae	9 g
Folium Nelumbinis	9 g
Radix Platycodi	9 g
Semen Lepiddii seu Descurainiae	9 g
Radix Angelicae Sinensis	9 g
Rhizoma seu Radix Notopterygii	6 g

Administration: Decoct the above drugs in water for oral dose. One dose daily.

2. Other Therapies

(1) Folium Mori 9 g
　　Flos Chrysanthemi 9 g
　　Borax 3 g
　　Chalcanthitum 3 g

Administration: Decoct the drugs in water. Use the decoction as an eye lotion to wash the eyes.

(2) Apply 10—50% eye droping of *Qianliguang* (89) drops to the eye.

(3) Acupuncture treatment: Needle the acupoints of Taiyang, Sibai, Quchi, Hegu with strong stimulation.

(4) Pricking for blood letting out: Select three of the posterior auricular veins or the points of Jiaosun, Taiyang, Erjian. After routine disinfection, prick any of the veins or any of the points with a three—edged needle to let off three drops of blood, one prick a time, once daily.

7.3 Acute Epidemic Conjunctivitis

Acute epidemic conjunctivitis is characterized by acute onset and high infectiousness, edema and congestion of the bulbar conjunctiva. It is caused by enterovirus or adenovirus. It is termed *Tian Xing Chiyan* in TCM.

Etiology and Pathogenesis

The disease is due to affection of epidemic pathogenic factors which travel upward along the lung channel and attack the eyes. If the epidemic pathogenic factors attack the eyes directly, or, if they combine with excessive heat of the lung and stomach and then jointly attack the eye, the disease will also occur.

Clinical Manifestations

There are photophobia and lacrimation, headache, pain of the orbit, red swollen eyelid, congestion and edema of bulbar conjunctiva, petechial or patchy subconjunctival hemorrhage. The eye secretion is mucous and comparatively scanty. There is spotted infiltration on the superficial layer of the cornea, which are absorbed slowly. The lymphoglandulae auriculares anteriores are swollen.

Type and Treatment

1. Internal Treatment

(1) Type of invasion of epidemic pathogenic factors.

Symptoms and signs: Photophobia, lacrimation, foreign body sensation, congestion and edema of the bulbar conjunctiva, headache, pain of the orbid, aversion to wind, lassitude, floating pulse, reddened tongue with thin, whitish coating.

Therapeutic Method: Expelling wind and epidemic pathogenic factors, clearing away heat and toxic material.

Recipe: Modified *Puji Xiaodu Yin* (31)

Ingredients:

Radix Isatidis	30 g
Lasiosphaera seu Calvatia	9 g
Fructus Arctii	9 g
Herba Menthae	9 g
Flos Chrysanthemi	9 g
Radix Bupleuri	9 g
Radix Platycodi	9 g
Cortex Mori Radicis	9 g
Fructus Forsythiae	15 g
Rhizoma Coptidis	6 g
Radix Scutellariae	9 g
Rhizoma Smilacis Glabrae	15 g
Radix Glycyrrhizae	9 g

Administration: Decoct the above drugs in water for oral dose. One dose daily.

(2) Type of excessiveness of noxious heat.

Symptoms and Signs: Photophobia, lacrimation, epiphora with hot sensation, edema of the eyelid, marked congestion and edema of the bulbar conjunctiva, subconjunctiva hemorrhage, preauricular lymphodeno swelling with tenderness, thirst with desire for drink, constipation, full and forceful pulse, reddened tongue with dry and yellow fur.

Therapeutic Method: Clearing away heat and toxic materials and expelling epidemic pathogenic factor.

Recipe: Modified *Qingwen Baidu Yin* (29)

Ingredients:

Gypsum Fibrosum	30 g
Rhizoma Anemarrhenae	9 g
Radix Glycyrrhizae	9 g
Rhizoma Coptidis	9 g
Radix Scutellariae	9 g
Fructus Gardeniae	9 g
Fructus Forsythiae	12 g
Radix Paeoniae Rubra	9 g
Cortex Moutan Radicis	9 g
Radix Rehmanniae	12 g
Radix Platycodi	9 g
Rhizoma Paridis	15 g
Folium Isatidis	6 g
Herba Menthae	9 g

Administration: Decoct the above drugs in water for oral dose. One dose daily.

2. Other Therapies

(1) Apply eye drop of 1% huangginsui (90) drops to the eye.

(2) Decoct 15 g Radix Isatidis or Folium Isatidis in water

and filtrate the decoction. Wash the eyes with the filtrated decoction.

(3) Pricking for blood letting out.

Select three of the posterior auricular veins. After routine disinfection, prick them with a three-edged needle to let five drops of blood out, once a day.

7.4 Chronic Catarrhal Conjunctivitis

The disease is characterized by dryness, foreign body sensation, itching in the eyes and slight congestion of the palpebral conjunctiva. It is a protracted and obstinate disease. The disease is usually caused by microorganic infection and irritation of chemical or physical agents. It is termed *Baise Zheng* in TCM.

Etiology and Pathogenesis

If a person suffers from deficiency of lung-*Yin*, the result will be hyperactivity of endogenous fire in the lung that impaires the purifying and descending function of this organ. When this is worsened by invasion of exogenous pathogenic wind and heat, the pathogens will flare up to attack the eye in collaboration with the endogenous deficiency-fire, and the disease occurs. Residens of previous intensive phathogenic wind and heat may incubate in the lung and spleen collaterals and when certain situation favowrable for them to proliferate exist, they will also cause the disease by flare up to attack the eye. Besides, excessive endogenous dampness and heat of the spleen and stomach will hinder refined essence of food from being sent to the upper organs. Retention of dampness and heat steaming-burning the eye and malnutrition of it will then lead to the disease.

Clinical Manifestations

Itching in both eyes, foreign body sensation, dry and burning sensation, desire for keeping the eyes closed, white frothy secretion at the lateral canthi, slight congestion of the palpebral conjunctiva, papillary hypertrophy of the palpebral conjunctiva with a velvet−like rough appearance.

Type and Treatment

1. Internal Treatment

(1) Type of insufficiency of lung−*Yin* and affection of exogenous wind−heat.

Symptoms and Signs: Dryness and discomfort of the eyes, itching with little secretion, slight photophobia and lacrimation, slight congestion of the palpebral conjunctiva, dry throat and mouth, floating and small pulse, reddened tongue with thin white coating.

Therapeutic Method: Nourishing *Yin* and clearing the lung heat, dispelling wind and heat.

Recipe: Modified *Sangbaipi Tang* (30)

Ingredients:

Cortex Mori Radicis	12 g
Radix Ophiopogonis	9 g
Radix Scrophulariae	9 g
Cortex Lycii Radicis	12 g
Radix Scutellariae	9 g
Flos Inulae	9 g
Flos Chrysanthemi	9 g
Radix Platycodi	9 g
Folium Nelumbinis	9 g
Radix Sophorae Subprostratae	9 g
Radix Trichosanthis	12 g

Radix Ledebouriellae　　9 g
Radix Glycyrrhizae　　9 g

Administration: Decoct the above drugs in water for oral dose. One dose daily. (The Folium Nelumbinis should be wrapped in gauze.)

(2) Type of accumulation of damp-heat.

Symptoms and Signs: Discomfort and burning sensation of the eyes, photophobia and lacrimation, congestion of the palpebral conjunctiva, papillary hypertrophy, slight congestion of the bulbar conjunctiva, dark yellow urine, soft and rapid pulse, reddened tongue with yellow and sticky coating.

Therapuetic Method: Clearing away heat, promoting diuresis and improving the dispersing function of the lung.

Recipe: Modified *Sanren Tang* (8)

Ingredients:

Talcum	30 g
Rhizoma Pinelliae	9 g
Semen Armeniacae Amarum	6 g
Semen Coicis	15 g
Semen Amomi Carddmomi	9 g
Herba Lophatheri	9 g
Cortex Mori Radicis	9 g
Rhizoma Alismatis	9 g
Poria Rubra	9 g
Radix Paeoniae Rubra	9 g

Administration: Decoct the above drugs in water for oral dose. Once a day.

(3) Type of incubation of residual pathogenic factor.

Symptoms and Signs: Dry and discomfortable sensation in

the eyes, slight burning sensation which gets severe in the afternoon or at night, itching, little secretion, slight congestion of the palpebral conjunctiva, dry cough and sore throat, floating and slightly rapid pulse, reddened tougne with thin and yellow coating.

Therapeutic Method: Clearing away insidious pathogenic heat in the lung channel.

Recipe: Modified *Xiefei Tang* (31)

Ingredients:

Cortex Mori Radicis	15 g
Radix Ophiopogonis	12 g
Cortex Lycii Radicis	9 g
Radix Scutellariae	9 g
Rhizoma Anemarrhenae	9 g
Radix Platycodi	9 g
Herba Menthae	9 g
Flos Chrysanthemi	9 g
Bulbus Fritillariae Thunbergii	9 g
Fructus Forsythiae	9 g
Radix Angelicae Sinensis Praeparata	12 g
Radix Glycyrrhizae	9 g

Administration: Decoct the above drugs in water for oral dose, once a day.

2. Other Therapies

(1) Cortex Mori Radicis　　　　　　　　　　9 g
　　Flos Chrysanthemi Albus　　　　　　　9 g

Decoct them in water and wash the eyes with the dicoction.

(2) Apply *Xihuang San* (91) to the eyes.

7.5 Phlyctenular Conjunctivitis

It is a circumscribed inflammation of the bulbar conjunctiva. It is a delayed allergy of the conjunctival epithelial tissue to certain sensitizing toxin. It is usually seen in the children with general asthenia. It is termed *Jingan* in TCM.

Etiology and Pathogensis

It is caused by obstruction of the vessels resulting from dysfunction of the lung as a consequence of accumulation of dryness and heat due to invasion of the lung by dryness which stagnates and consequently produces heat. Besides, if a patient with constant deficiency of lung—*Yin* is attacked by exogenous dryness, he will suffer severer insufficiency of *Yin*. This may then cause asthenic fire to flare up and give rise to obstruction of the channels and vessels. Consequently, the disease occurs.

Clinical Manifestations

There is foreign body sensation, slight pain and itching, photophobia and lacrimation. Grayish—white phlyctenule can be seen in the bulbar conjunctiva or in the limbus cornea. The phlyctenule is surrounded by localized hyperemia.

Type and Treatment

1. Internal Treatment

(1) Type of accumulation of dryness and heat.

Symptoms and Signs: There is foreign body sensation, slight pain, photophobia and lacrimation. Pinkish white phlyctenule can be seen on the bulbar conjunctiva, which is surrounded by localized hyperemia. The other symptoms in clude thirst, dryness of mouth, little rapid pulse, dry and reddened tongue with thin and yellow coating.

Therapeutic Method: Moistening the lung and removing obstruction, removing pathogenic heat and cooling the blood.

Recipe Modified *Qingzao Jiufei Tang* (32)

Ingredients:

Gypsum Fibrosum	30 g
Rhizoma Anemarrhenae	9 g
Folium Mori	9 g
Semen Armeniacae Amarum	3 g
Folium Eriobotryae	9 g
Radix Ophiopogonis	12 g
Fructus Trichosanthis	12 g
Fructus Cannabis	12 g
Cortex Moutan Radicis	9 g
Radix Paeoniae Rubra	9 g
Bulbus Lylii Praeparata	9 g
Radix Glycyrrhizae	9 g

Administration: Decoct the above drugs in water for oral dose, once a day.

(2) Type of lingering of pathogens due to *Yin* deficiency.

Symptoms and Signs: The eye symptoms are the same as those of the last type. The disease recurs repeatedly, accompained with dry mouth and throat, dry cough, thready pulse, reddened tongue with little coating.

Therapeutic Method: Nourishing *Yin* to moisten dryness, promoting the dispersing function of the lung to eliminate pathogenic heat.

Recipe: Modified *Yejin Tang* (33)

Ingredients:

Radix Scrophulariae	12 g

Cortex Mori Radicis	9 g
Semen Armeniacae Amarum	3 g
Rhizoma Coptidis	9 g
Radix Scutellariae	9 g
Semen Lepiddii seu Descurainiae	12 g
Radix Arichosanthis	12 g
Flos Chrysanthemi	9 g
Radix Ledebouriellae	9 g
Fructus Aurantii	9 g
Radix Platycodi	12 g
Radix Glycyrrhizae	9 g

Administration: Decoct the above drugs in water for oral dose, once a day.

2. Other Therapies

(1) Flos Carthami	9 g
Flos Lonicerae	30 g
Retinervus Luffae Fructus	9 g

Decoct them in water and wash the eyes with the decoction, three times a day.

(2) Auriculo-acupuncture.

Needle the points Endocrine, Eye, Jiaogan, and Shenmen once a day. Twist the needles once every fives minutes, and retain the needles for twenty minutes.

7.6 Spring Catarrhal Conjunctivitis

The disease is an interstitial proliferating inflammation of the conjunctiva with special morphology. It is caused by hypersensitivity. Cilniically the disease can be divided into palpebral conjunctival type, bulbar conjunctival type and mix type. The characteristic feature of it is that the patients' condition gets worse during spring and summer and relieved spontaneously in autumn and winter but recurs in next spring. The allergens are usually of physical factors. In TCM, it is termed *"Mu-yang"* or *"Shifu Zheng"*.

Etiology and Pathogenesis

When retention of dampness and heat in the spreen channel and stagnation of seasonal intensive exogenous wind and heat in the lung combine with each other they tend to go upward to attack the eye, the eyelid and the conjunctiva and the disease will occur. Besides, defeciency of blood, a condition that will result in endogenouse wind, frequently makes the patient susceptible to invasion of exogenous pathogenic wind. When the endogenous wind attacks the eye in collaboration with the exogenous wind, the disease occurs.

Clinical Manifestations

Intense itching of the eyes, burning and foreign body sensation, photophobia, lacrimation, thick ropy secretion, plus marked congestion of the palpebral conjunctiva, with hard and flattened papillae in different sizes all over the palpebral conjunctiva giving an appearance of oval stone road surface, or plus bulbar conjunctival congestion, pigmentation in a turbid, yellowish-red color and grayish-yellow colloid pachynsis at the corneal imbus, or plus both of the conditions described above.

Type and Treatment

1. Internal Treatment

(1) Type of Dampness-heat in the spleen channel in combination with attack of exogenous wind-heat.

Symptoms and Signs: Beside all the symptoms described in

clinical manifestations the patient may have somnolence, greasy mouth, anorexia, floating pulse, and reddened tongue with greasy, yellowish coating.

Therapeutic Method: Clearing away heat, promoting diuresis, dispelling wind and arresting itching.

Recipe: Modified *Xiaofeng Chure Tang* (34)

Ingredients:

Radix Scutellariae	9 g
Fructus Gardeniae	9 g
Cortex Fraxini	9 g
Radix Bupleuri	12 g
Radix Peucedani	9 g
Radix Ledebouriellae	9 g
Radix Angelicae Dahuricae	9 g
Herba Menthae	12 g
Radix et Rhizoma Rhei	3 g
Radix Sophorae Flavescentis	12 g
Radix Puerariae	12 g
Gypsum Fibrosum	15 g
Radix Cynanchi Paniculati	30 g
Radix Glycyrrhizae	9 g

Administration: Decoct the above drugs in water for oral dose. One dose daily.

(2) Type of attack of pathogenic wind due to deficiency of blood.

Symptoms and Signs: Intense itching, unbearable dryness, foreign body sensation, photophobia lacrimation which gets severe when the eyes are facing the wind, congestion of palpebral conjunctiva, blurred vessels, slight bulbar conjunctiva congestion in turbid color, pallid complxion, wearines and lassitude, deep and thready pulse, pink tongue with little coating.

Therapeutic Method: Nourishing the blood, expelling wind, promoting blood circulation and alleviating itching.

Recipe: Modified *Danggui Huoxue Yin* (35)
Ingredients:

Radix Angelicae Sinensis	15 g
Radix Rehmanniae Praeparata	9 g
Radix Paeoniae Alba	15 g
Rhizoma Ligustici Chuanxiong	9 g
Rhizoma seu Radix Notopterygii	9 g
Herba Menthae	9 g
Radix Ledebouriellae	9 g
Radix Paeoniae Rubra	9 g
Radix Astrahalis seu Hedysari	15 g
Rhizoma Atractylodis	9 g
Radix Glycyrrhizae	9 g
Poria	12 g
Radix Codonopsis Pilosulae	9 g

Administration: Decoct the above drugs in water for oral dose. One dose daily.

2. Other Therapies

(1) Apply *Chunxue Gao* (92) to the eye, three times a day.

(2) Acupuncture: Needle the acupoints Jingming, Taiyang, Hegu and Zusanli, with medium stimulation. Once a day.

7.7 Pterygium

Pterygium is formed by degeneration and proliferation of the epithelial tissue of the bulbar conjunctiva. It is a triangular fold of mucous membrane, expanding from the inner or outer part of the ocular conjunctiva toward the cornea, mostly at the palpebral fissure. It can be classified into progressive type and stationary type. It is termed *Nurou Panjing* in TCM.

Etiology and Pathogenesis

When the patient suffers from hyperactive heat-fire, endogenous wind will arise from it, Then the fire and wind may reinforce each other and go upward to attack the canthi, causing the disease. Besides, invasion of exogenous wind and heat may first affect the lung and the consequent wind-heat in the lung channel may then go upward to attack the inner canthi. Hance the disease.

Clinical Manifestations

Dryness, foreign body sensation with itching of the eyes, congestion and thickening of the bulbar conjunctiva usually in the inner side of the palpebral fissure, presenting a triangular shape expanding toward the cornea. The pterygium can be divided into three parts: the head, the neck and the body. If the head is a sharp grayish-white colloid projection and the neck and the body are scarcoid and congested with thickening tissue, the pterygium is progressive. If the head is flat and the blood vessels of the neck and body are contracted with thin tissue, the pterygium is stationary.

Type and Treatment

1. Internal Treatment

(1) Type of flaming of the heart fire.

Symptoms and Signs: Xenophthalmia and discomfort, congestion and thickening of the pterygium, caked secretion, dysphoria, thirst, aphthae, scanty and dark urine, rapid pulse, reddened tip of the tongue with yellow fur.

Therapeutic Method: Clearing away heart fire, removing heat from the blood and dissipating blood stasis.

Recipe: Modified *Xiexin Tang* (36)

Ingredients:

Rhizoma Coptidis	9 g
Fructus Forsythiae	15 g
Plumula Nelumbinis	3 g
Herba Lophatheri	12 g
Radix Glycyrrhizae	12 g
Radix Rehmanniae	9 g
Radix Paeoniae Rubra	9 g
Radix Angelicae Sinensis	9 g
Fructus Leonuri	12 g
Gypsum Fibrosum	30 g
Spica Schizonepetae	9 g
Radix Ledebouriellae	9 g
Radix Curcumae	9 g

Administration: Decoct the above drugs in water for oral dose. Once a day.

(2) Wind-heat in the lung channel.

Symptoms and Signs: There is xenophthalmia and itching in the eyes. Progressing quickly the pterygium is red, and its head is sharp and projected. Other symptoms include dry throat and coughing, floating and rapid pulse, reddened tongue with thin and yellow coating.

Therapeutic Method: Ventilating the lung, dispelling wind, clearing away heat and activating collaterals.

Recipe: Modified *Xiefei Yin* (27)

Ingredients:

Radix Scutellariae	9 g
Cortex Mori Radicis	9 g
Cortex Lycii Radicis	9 g
Fructus Gardeniae	12 g
Fructus Forsythiae	15 g
Caulis Akebiae	6 g
Radix Glycyrrhizae	9 g
Herba Menthae	9 g
Flos Chrysanthemi	12 g
Radix Ledebouriellae	9 g
Radix Rehmanniae	12 g
Radix Scrophulariae	9 g
Cortex Moutan Radicis	9 g

Administration: Decoct the above drugs in water for oral dose. One dose daily.

(3) Type of hyperactivity of fire due to *Yin* deficiency.

Symptoms and Signs: The pterygium is pink in color with a flat head. There is distress in the chest, dire thirst, deep and thready pulse, reddened tongue with little coating.

Therapeutic Method: Nourishing *Yin* and reducing pathogenic fire

Recipe: Modified *Ziyin Jianghuo Tang* (37)

Ingredients:

Radix Rehmanniae	12 g
Radix Ophiopogonis	9 g
Rhizoma Anemarrhenae	9 g
Cortex Phellodendri	6 g
Radix Scutellariae	9 g

Radix Angelicae Sinensis	9 g
Rhizoma Rehmanniae Praeparatae	9 g
Radix Paeoniae Alba	12 g
Radix Glycyrrhizae	9 g
Radix Bupleuri	9 g
Herba Lycopi	9 g
Radix Adenophorae Strictae	9 g

Administration: Decoct the above drugs in water for oral dose. One dose daily.

2. Other Therapies

Excision should be made if neccessary.

8 Diseases of the Sclera

The function of the sclera is to protect the intraocular contents. The sclera falls into the category of the white of the eye in TCM, corresponding to the lung and belonging to *Qi* orbiculus. Therefore, diseases of the sclera have a close relationship with the lung. In treatment, such methods as clearing away heat, moistening the lung, ventilating the lung and eliminating the pathogenic factors are mainly used.

8.1 Scleritis

According to the location and depth of the lesion, the disease can be classified into episcleritis and Scleritis. In severe cases it may give rise to complications in the cornea and uvea. The main etiology is attributed to endogenous factors basically under the category of collagenous diseases. In TCM it is termed *Huo Gan*.

Etiology and Pathogenesis

In a person, accumulation of excessive lung–heat always leads to dysfunction of the lung in dispersing and desending and to disorder of *Qi*–flow, causing stagnation of *Qi* and blood stass. If vessels and channel of the white of the eye are obstructed by the stagnation and stass, the disease will occur. Apart from this, hyperactive heat–fire tends to burn the lung firstly and then, the white of the eye will be diseased. Sometimes, excessivs endogenous dampness and heat may be stired by invasion of endogenous pathogenous wind, and then, the wind will go upward together with the dampness and heat to attack the eye, causing obstruction of vessels and channels there. Hence the disease occurs.

Clinical Manifestations

Foreign body sensation, photophobia, lacrimation, pain of the eyeball which gets severe at night, localized congestion of sclera in violet red or purplish—blue color, nodular or slightly diffuse projections with tenderness and inflammation involving the cornea and iris.

Type and Treatment

1. Internal Treatment

(1) Type of excessiveness of the lung—heat.

Symptoms and signs: There are photophobia, lacrimation, pain of the eyeball, episcleral congestion in violet—red color, nodular projection, dry mouth and sore throat, cough, rapid pulse, reddened tongue with thin and yellowish coating.

Therapeutic Method: Clearing away heat and improving the dispersing function of the lung, promoting blood circulation and removing obstruction of the channels.

Recipe: Modified *Sangbaipi Tang* (30)

Ingredients:

Cortex Mori Radicis	15 g
Radix Ophiopogonis	9 g
Radix Scrophulariae	9 g
Cortex Lycii Radicis	12 g
Radix Scutellariae	9 g
Flos Chrysanthemi	9 g
Radix Platycodi	9 g
Semen Lepiddii seu Descurainiae	9 g

Herba Menthae	9 g
Fructus Arctii	12 g
Bulbus Fritillariae Thunbergii	9 g
Radix Paeoniae Rubra	9 g
Flos Carthami	9 g
Spica Prunellae	15 g

Administration: Decoct the above drugs in the water for oral dose. One dose daily.

(2) Type of hyperactive heart—fire.

Symptoms and signs: Photophobia, lacrimation, distending pain of the eyeball, scleral congestion in purplish dark color, localized diffuse projection, aphthae, scanty and dark urine, slightly rapid pulse, reddened tip of the tongue, and thin and yellowish coating.

Therapeutic Method: Clearing away the heart fire, removing heat from the blood and eliminating obstruction of the channels.

Recipe: Modified *Xiexin Tang* (36)

Ingredients:

Rhizoma Coptidis	9 g
Fructus Forsythiae	12 g
Radix Rehmanniae	12 g
Radix Peaoniae Rubra	9 g
Herba Lophatheri	9 g
Radix Glycyrrhizae	9 g
Radix et Rhizoma Rhei	3 g
Caulis Akebiae	9 g
Resina Boswelliae Carterii Praeparata	9 g
Resina Commiphorae Myrrhae Praeparata	9 g
Lignum Sappan	9 g

Spina Gleditsiae	9 g

Administration: Decoct the above drugs in water for oral dose. One dose daily.

(3) Type of attack of pathogenic wind, dampness and heat.

Symptoms and signs: Photophobia, acrimation, scleral congestion in dark red color, headache, oppressed feeling in chest, arthralgia, slippery pulse, slightly reddened tongue with thick and white coating.

Therapeutic Method: Expelling the wind, eliminating dampness, clearing away heat and removing obstruction of the channels.

Recipe: Modfied *Sanfeng Chushi Huoxue Tang* (38)
Ingredients:

Rhizoma seu Radix Notopterygii	9 g
Radix Angelicae Pubescentis	9 g
Radix Ledebouriellae	9 g
Radix Peucedani	12 g
Rhizoma Atractylodis Macrocephalae	9 g
Caulis Lonicerae	15 g
Radix Angelicae Sinensis	9 g
Radix Paeoniae Rubra	12 g
Caulis Spatholobi	30 g
Flos Carthami	9 g
Poria Rubra	9 g
Fructus Aurantii	9 g
Radix Platycodi	9 g
Radix Glycyrrhizae	9 g

Administration: Decoct the above drugs in water for oral dose. One dose daily.

2. Other therapies
(1) Apply *Wudan Gao* (93) to the eye.
(2) Point injection therapy:
   Inject 0.25 ml of 0.5% procaine into each of the points: Tongziliao, Jingming, Sibai, Yuyao, once a day.
(3) Propietary: *Yangyin Qingfei Wan* (107)
   Administration: 9 g each time, three times daily.

9 Corneal Diseases

Corneal diseases are characterized by: (1) slow repairment of the lesion and long course of the illness because, with poor nourishment due to lack of vessels in this tissue, metablolism in the corneal is very slow; (2) varying degree of impairment to the visual function because there may be some residual scar of opacity left on the transparent cornael after recovery from the disease.

In terms of five orbiculi the cornea is wind orbiculus, which corresponds to the liver in the interior of the body. The liver and the gallbladder are interior—exteriorly related. So type differentiation and treatment of corneal diseases begins with analysis of the condition of the liver and the gallbladder. At early stage, the diseases mostly fall into type of wind—heat, or heat of excess type of the liver channel; At late stage the diseases may recur repeatedly or they may be chronic with remissions and exacerbations, falling into type of deficiency of the liver *Yin*. During the treatment, in addition to prescriptions based on type differentiation, drugs for removing nebula should be used if necessary so as to promote restoration of visual function.

9.1 Serpiginous Corneal Ulcer

It is a suppurative corneal ulcer, which is usually caused by the infection of pneumococci, staphylococci, etc. The ulcer usually spreads into the center of the cornea, accompanied by hypopyon. So it is also called hypopyon corneal ulcer and termed

Ning Zhi Yi in TCM.

Etiology and Pathogenesis

The disease may be due to trauma of the corneal superficies followed by invasion of exogenouse wind and heat, or due to formation of pus on the corneal, a consequent condition following *Qi* stagnation and blood stasis caused by hyperactive fire of the liver and gallbladder that goes upward to attack the eye. It may also envolve from keratitis of other type that is worsened by invasion of exogenous pathogenic factors.

Clinical Manifestations

Foreign body sensation and pain in the eyes, ophthalmalgia, photophobia, lacrimation and blurred vision. Clinical examination shows ciliary congestion or mixed congestion. At the initial stage there are greyish white spots of infiltration in the center of cornea, which may spread both in area and depth to form ulcer. Because the iris is irritated, cloudy agueous and hypopyon will occur. In severe cases, the corneal ulcer may spread deeper resulting in perforation. Most cases will recover by forming leukoma adhaerens, but in a few severe cases, corneal staphyloma, endophthalmitis, or panophthalmitis may be induced, leading to blindness and atrophy of the eyeball.

Type and Treatment

1. Internal Treatment

(1) Type of excessiveness of wind-heat.

Symptoms and Signs: At the initial stage the patient complains of slight foreign body sensation in the eyes, photophobia, lacrimation and hypopsia, ciliary congestion, infiltrations in the centre of the cornea, other symptoms include headache, reddened tongue with thin and whitish or yellowish fur, and floating, rapid pulses.

Therapeutic Method: Dispelling wind and removing heat.

Recipe: Modified *Xinzhi Chailian Tang* (39)

Ingredients:

Radix Bupleuri	9 g
Fructus Viticis	9 g
Herba Schizonepetae	9 g
Radix Ledebouriellae	9 g
Radix Scutellariae	9 g
Fructus Gardeniae	9 g
Radix Gentianae	9 g
Caulis Akebiae	6 g
Herba Equiseti Hiemalis	12 g
Radix Paeoniae Rubra	15 g
Radix Glycyrrhizae	6 g

Administration: Decoct the above drugs in water for oral dose, once a day.

(2) Type of hyperactivity of fire in the liver and the gallbladder.

Symptoms and Signs: Ophthalmalgia, photophobia, lacrimation, obvious exacerbation of blurred vision, mixed congestion, corneal ulcer, hypopyon, accompanied by dry mouth and throat, constipation, deep-colored urine, reddened tongue with yellowish fur, wiry and rapid pulse.

Therapeutic Method: Clearing away liver-fire.

Recipe: Modified *Longdan Xiegan Tang* (40)

Ingredients:

Radix Gentianae	9 g
Fructus Gardeniae	9 g

Radix Scutellariae	9 g
Radix Bupleuri	9 g
Rhizoma Alismatis	9 g
Caulis Akebiae	9 g
Semen Plantaginis	9 g
Radix Rehmanniae	15 g
Radix Angelicae Sinensis	12 g
Flos Eriocauli	12 g

Administration: Decoct the above drugs in water for oral dose. One dose daily.

Modification: for cases with oppilation add:

Radix et Rhizoma Rhei	9 g
Nalrii Sulfas	9 g

for cases with dysphoria and thirst, add:

Gypsum Fibrosum	15 g
Rhizoma Anemarrhenae	9 g

for cases with sever opthalmagia, add:

Radix Paeoniae Rubra	15 g
Flos Carthami	9 g

(3) Type of weakened body resistance and ligering pathogenic factors.

Symptoms and signs: The symptoms are relieved and corneal ulcer is partially repaired. The course is usually long and the condition of the patient is mild but chronic. The tongue is pale and the pulse is faint.

Therapeutic Method: Strengthening the body resistance and eliminating pathogenic factors.

Recipe: Modified *Tuolixiaodu San* (41)

Ingredients:

Radix Astragali seu Hedysari	30 g
Rhizoma Ligustici Chuanxiong	9 g
Radix Angelicae Sinensis	12 g
Rhizoma Atractylodis Macrocephalae	12 g
Poria	12 g
Radix Ginseng	12 g
Flos Lonicerae	18 g
Radix Angelicae Dahuricae	9 g
Radix Platycodi	9 g
Periostracum Cicadae	9 g
Flos Eriocauli	15 g
Fructus Tribuli	15 g

Administration: Decoct the above drugs in water for oral dose.

2. Other Therapies

(1) 10% eye drops of Herba Senecionis Scandentis (89), or 10% eye drops of Rhizoma Coptidis (94) may be instilled in the eye once every one to two hours.

(2) 0.5 ml of *Yin Huang* injection (95) may be injected under the bulbar conjunctiva once a day.

(3) Mydriatic may be instilled.

(4) *Tuiyun San* (98) may be used at the late stage once a day.

9.2 Herpes Simplex Keratitis

Herpes simplex keratitis is a common corneal disease. The incidence of the disease has increased obviously in recent years. It is caused by direct infection of virus of herpes febrilis in the corneal epithelial cells. The affection is generally unilateral and it may affect people of all ages. It is analogous to *Juxing Zhang* in

TCM.

Etiology and Pathogenesis

When a person with hyperactive liver fire is exposed to invasion of exogenous pathogenic wind and heat, the endogenous fire will combine with the intensive pathogens and go upward together to attack the eye, causing the disease. Besides, accumulation of dampness and heat in the spleen and stomach due to improper diet, or flaming up of asthenic fire resulting from deficiency of liver—*Yin* and kidney—*Yin* may also lead to the disease.

Clinical Manifestations

There is a history of fever due to infection of the upper respiratory tract before the attack of the disease. The patient complains of slight foreign body sensation, photophobia, lacrimation, and blurred vision. There is ciliary congestion, greyish white punctate infiltrations in the corneal superficial layer which are later confluent and become dendritic. The infiltration may expand both in width and in depth to form map—like superficial ulcer with irregular margins. If the corneal propria is involved, the disease may be complicated with iritis.

Type and Treatment

1. Internal Treatment

(1) Type of wind—heat of the liver channel.

Symptoms and Signs: There is a foreign body sensation, photophobia, lacrimation, divergent greyish white punctate infiltrations on the cornea, accompanied with fever, aversion to cold, thin and yellowish fur, and floating and rapid pulse.

Therapeutic Method: Dispelling wind and removing heat

Recipe: Modified *Qianghuo Shengfeng Tang* (42)

Ingredients:

Radix Bupleuri	9 g
Herba Schizonepetae	9 g
Radix Ledebouriellae	9 g
Radix Peucedani	9 g
Rhizoma seu Radix Notopterygii	9 g
Radix Angelicae Pubescentis	9 g
Herba Menthae	9 g
Rhizoma Ligustici Chuanxiong	9 g
Radix Angelicae Dahuricae	9 g
Radix Scutellariae	9 g
Fructus Aurantii	9 g
Radix platycodi	9 g
Rhizoma Atractylodis Macrocephalae	12 g
Radix Glycyrrhizae	6 g

Administration: Decoct the above drugs in water for oral dose.

(2) Type of hyperactivity of fire of the liver.

Symptoms and Signs: The eye symptoms are aggravated distinctly with blurred vision. The corneal infiltration may expand and become deeper, accompanied with headache, dark colored urine, yellow fur, and wiry, rapid pulse.

Therapeutic Method: Purging the liver of the pathogenic fire.

Recipe: Modified *Longdan Xiegan Tang* (40)

Ingredients:

Radix Gentianae	9 g
Fructus Gardeniae	9 g
Radix Scutellariae	9 g
Radix Bupleuri	9 g
Caulis Akebiae	9 g

Rhizoma Alimatis	9 g
Radix Rehmanniae	15 g
Flos Buddejae	30 g
Herba Equiseti Hiemalis	12 g
Radix Paeoniae Rubra	15 g

Administration: Decoct the above drugs in water for oral dose.

(3) Type of retention of endogenous dampness and heat.

Symptoms and Signs: Chronic and obstinate inflammation of the cornea, heaviness in the head, oppressed feeling in the chest, yellowish urine and loose stools, stickness of the mouth, reddened tongue with yellowish and greasy fur, and floating pulse.

Therapeutic Method: Removing dampness and heat.

Recipe: Modified *Sanren Tang* (8)

Ingredients:

Semen Armeniacae Amarum	9 g
Semen Coicis	9 g
Rhizoma Pinelliae	9 g
Cortex Magnoliae Officinalis	9 g
Herba Lophathari	9 g
Talcum	9 g
Flos Lonicerae	18 g
Herba Taraxaci	30 g
Periostracum Cicadae	9 g
Radix Glycyrrhizae	6 g

Administration: Decoct the above drugs in water for oral dose. once a day.

(4) Type of hyperactivity of endogenous fire due to *Yin* defi-

ciency.

Symptoms and Signs: Slight but chronic and obstinate inflammation of the cornea, reddened tongue with little coating, small and rapid pulse.

Therapeutic Method: Nourishing *Yin* and clearing away heat.

Recipe: Modified *Zhibai Dihuang Tang* (43)

Ingredients:

Rhizoma Anemarrhenae	9 g
Cortex Phellodendri	9 g
Rhizoma Alismatis	9 g
Rhizoma Dioscoreae	9 g
Poria	12 g
Radix Rehmanniae	12 g
Semen Cassiae	12 g
Flos Eriocauli	12 g
Radix Scrophulariae	15 g

Administration: Decoct the above drugs in water for oral dose. once a day.

2. Other Therapies

(1) 10% eye drops of Herba Andrographitis (96) or 10% eye drops of Herba Senecionis Scandentis (89) can be applied to the eye.

(2) Decoct Flos Lonicerae, Folium Mori, Flos Chrysanthemi Indici, Radix Ledebouriellae Herba Taraxaci in water. Filtrat the decoction and use it for eye-rinsing or for hot compresses.

(3) *Tuiyun San* (98) should be used to remove the nebula at the late stage of the disease.

(4) Acupuncture Treatment: The commonly used points are

Jingming, Sibai, Chengqi, Sizhukong, Hegu, Guangming, Zusanli, etc. Needle 3 local points and 2 distal points, once a day.

(5) Proprietary: *Huanglian Shangqing Wan* (102) for oral administration, one bolus a time twice daily.

9.3 Deep Keratitis

Deep keratitis is characterized by irregular infiltration and hydrops in the corneal stroma layer. It may be caused by viral infection, or by some allergic factors. It is termed *Hunjing Zhang* in TCM.

Etiology and Pathogenesis

It is usually due to wind—heat of the liver channel or excessiveness of pathogenic heat go upward to attack the eye; or it may also be caused by hyperactivity of endogenous fire due to deficiency of *Yin* resulting from protracted pathogens which consume *Yin* fluid.

Clinical Manifestations

Slight redness in the eye, photophobia, lacrimation, ophthalmalgia, blurred vision. Clinical examination will reveal ciliary congestion. The superficial layers of the cornea are smooth, while the stroma layer may present grayish white, glass—like opacity with indistinct margins, or discoid opacity with distinct margins. In the pathologic area the cornea is thickened, and the endothelia are edematous and rough. The disease may be complicated with iridocyclitis.

Type and Treatment

1. Internal Treatment

(1) Type of excessiveness of wind—heat.

Symptoms and Signs: Photophobia, lacrimation, mild

ophthalmalgia, blurred vision, ciliary congestion, misty opacity in deep layer of the cornea, accompanied by headache, fever, reddened tongue with thin whitish or yellowish fur, and floating, rapid pulse.

Therapeutic Method: Eliminating wind and clearing away heat.

Recipe: Modified *Sangju Yin* (44)

Ingredients:

Folium Mori	12 g
Flos Chrysanthemi	12 g
Rhizoma Phragmitis	12 g
Radix Platycodi	12 g
Fructus Forsythiae	9 g
Radix Ledebouriellae	9 g
Herba Menthae	9 g
Rhizoma Alismetis	9 g
Radix Paeoniae Rubra	15 g
Fructus Leonuri	15 g
Radix Glycyrrhizae	6 g

Administration: Decoct the above drugs in water for oral dose. One dose daily.

Modification: for cases with distinct hydrops add:

Semen Plantaginis	12 g
Semen Coicis	12 g

for cases at the late stage of the inflammation, add:

Semen Cassiae	12 g
Fructus Tribuli	12 g

(2) Type of dampness—heat of the liver and spleen.

Symptoms and Signs: Ophthalmalgia, exacerbation of

photophobia and lacrimation, accompanied by anorexia, halitosis, chest distress, constipation, reddened tongue with yellow and greasy fur, and rapid pulse.

Therapeutic Method: Clearing away heat and eliminating damp.

Recipe: Modified *Yinghau Jiedu Tang* (45)

Ingredients:

Flos Lonicerae	30 g
Herba Violae	15 g
Fructus Forsythiae	9 g
Radix Paeoniae Rubra	15 g
Spica Prunellae	12 g
Radix Rehmanniae	15 g
Cortex Moutan Radicis	9 g
Herba Agastachis	9 g
Rhizoma Pinelliae	9 g
Cortex Magnoliae Officinalis	9 g

Administration: Decoct the above drugs in water for oral dose.

(3) Type of hyperactivity of endogenous fire due to *Yin* deficiency.

Symptoms and Signs: The symptoms in the eyes are moderate but they recur repeatedly. The tongue is reddened with little fur, and the pulse is small and rarpid.

Therapeutic Method: Nourishing *Yin* and reducing pathogenic fire.

Recipe: Modified *Dabuyin Wan* (46)

Ingredients:

Rhizoma Anemarrhenae	9 g

Cortex Phellodendri	9 g
Cortex Moutan Radicis	9 g
Radix Rehmanniae Praeparata	15 g
Plastrum Testudinis	15 g
Radix Scrophulariae	15 g
Flos Buddlejae	18 g
Herba Equiseti Hiemalis	12 g
Radix Glycyrrhizae	6 g

Administration: Decoct the above drugs in water for oral dose, once a day.

2. Other Therapies

(1) Instill eyedrops of *Sanhuang Yanye* (97) in the eye, four times daily.

(2) Instill eye-drops of *Huanglian Xigua Shuang* (88), three times daily.

(3) Apply *Xihuang San* (91) to the eye at the late stage, three times daily.

(4) Apply 0.5% Liquid Atropin to the eye for those complicated by iritis, once a day.

(5) Propietary: *Lingqiao Jiedu Wan* or *Huanglian Shangqing Wan* for oral administration, 9 g a. time, twice a day.

9.4 Fascicular Keratitis

The disease is characterized by miliaria in the corneal superficial layer with a bundle of neogenetic blood vessels. It falls into anaphylactic keratitis, it mostly occurs in children with frequent recurrence. It is termed *Fenglun Chidou* in TCM.

Etiology and Pathogenesis

It is caused by stagnation of *Qi* and blood resulting from

dryness—heat of the liver channel, or by accumulation of mixture of phlegm and *Qi* resulting from deficiency of spleen—*Qi* that leads to phlegm—dampness.

Clinical Manifestations

At the initial stage there are grayish — white infiltrational spots in the corneal limbus, which look like herpes and may gradually stretche towards the centre. From the corneal limbus, a sheaf of newborn blood vessels spread into the margins of the infiltration and creep gradually towards the central area of the cornea. The herpes ruptured, producing ulcers. After recovery, it may leave circular cicatricial opacity, which may affect vision to a greater or lesser degree. The patient complains of ophthalmalgia, foreign body sensation, photophobia, lacrimation or blepharospasm.

Type and Treatment

1. Internal Treatment

(1)Type of accumlation of heat of the liver channel.

Symptoms and Signs: There is severe photophobia, lacrimation, foreign body sensation, ophthalmalgia, accompanied by a dry throat and a bitter taste in the mouth, reddened tongue with yellow fur, and wiry, rapid pulse.

Therapeutic Method: Purging the liver of pathogenic fire and clearing away heat

Recipe: Modified *Longdan Xiegan Tang* (40)

Ingredients:

Radix Gentianae	9 g
Radix Scutellariae	9 g
Fructus Gardeniae	9 g
Radix Bupleuri	9 g
Caulis Akebiae	9 g

Rhizoma Alismatis	9 g
Radix Rehmanniae	15 g
Radix Paeoniae Rubra	15 g
Semen Cassiae	12 g
Spica Prunellae	12 g

Administration: Decoct the above drugs in water for oral dose, once a day.

(2) Type of phlegm syndrome due to hypofunction of the spleen.

Symptoms and Signs: Mild eye symptoms, repeated recurrence accompanied by pallor complexion, hypodynamia of the extremities, pale tongue with thin fur, and weak pulse.

Therapeutic Method: Strengthening the spleen, replenishing Qi, reducing phlegm and resolving the mass.

Recipe: Modified *Xiangbei Yangrong Tang* (47)

Ingredients:

Radix Ginseng	12 g
Rhizoma Atractylodis Nacrocephalae	12 g
Radix Rehmanniae Praeparata	12 g
Radix Paeoniae Alba	12 g
Radix Angelicae Sinensis	12 g
Poria	9 g
Rhizoma Ligustici Chuanxiong	9 g
Radix Platycodi	9 g
Rhizoma Cyperi	9 g
Spica Prunellae	12 g
Semen Celosiae	12 g

Administration: Decoct the above drugs in water for oral dose, once a day.

2. Other therapies

(1) Instill eyedrops of *Sanhuang Yanye* (97), four to six times daily.

(2) Small amount of *Tuiyun San* (98) can be applied, three times daily.

(3) Antibiotic and hormone can be instilled in the eyes if necessary.

9.5 Keratomalacia

Keratomalacia is an ophthalmopathy caused by severe malnutrition mainly due to Vitamin A deficiency. The main symptom is sicca degeneration occurring in general skin, mucosa, conjunctiva and cornea. The disease may result in blindness. It mostly occurs in children and affects both eyes. It is termed *GanjiShangmu* in TCM.

Etiology and Pathogenesis

In infants, improper diet or feeding, food preference or weak constitution due to protracted illness will enfeeble the spleen and stomach, cause dysfunction of the spleen in transportation of refined essence and thus lead to malnutrition. In addition, if the child suffers from deficiency of liver—*Yin* and insufficiency of blood, he / she will become vulnerable to endogenous liver— heat and malnutrition of the eyes, and, then the disease occurs.

Clinical Manifestations

In early stage night blindness occurs and then the bulbar conjunctiva loses its normal lustre. Rugosity may occur when the eyeball turns to lateral sides. The cornea becomes dim and lusterless. As the condition gets drastic, triangular dry spots will occur in the bulbar conjunctiva of the palpebral fissure, and the cornea presents ground-glass-like opacity and its epithelium exfoliates. Secondary infection results in infiltration, ulceration, hypopyon and perforation of the ulcer, which finally leads to blindness.

Type and Treatment

1. Internal Treatment

(1) Type of deficiency of the spleen and the stomach.

Symptoms and Signs: At the early stage there is night blindness, lustreless bulbar conjunctiva and cornea, accompanied by abdominal distension, emaciation with sallow complexion, lassitude, hypodynamia, pale tongue with white and slightly thick fur, and sunken, weak pulse.

Therapeutic Method: Replenishing *Qi* and invigorating the spleen.

Recipe: Modified *Shenling Baishu San* (48)

Ingredients:

Radix Codonopsis Pilosulae	12 g
Rhizoma Atractylodis Macrocephalae	9 g
Poria	9 g
Radix Paeoniae Alba	9 g
Radix Angelicae Sinensis	9 g
Rhizoma Dioscoreae	9 g
Fructus Amomi	9 g
Pericarpium Citri Reticulatae	9 g
Radix Platycodi	9 g
Semen Dolichoris	9 g
Radix Glycyrrhizae	6 g

Administration: Decoct the above drugs in water for oral dose, once a day.

(2) Type of Liver heat due to hypofunction of the spleen.

Symptoms and Signs: Congested eye, photophobia, lacrimation, corneal opacity or ulcer, accompanied by abdominal distension, loose stools, afternoon hectic fever, restlessness, cloudy and greasy fur, and small, soft or small, wiry pulse.

Therapeutic Method: Invigorating the spleen, improving infantile malnutrition and clearing away liver−heat.

Recipe: Modified *Feier Wan* (49)
Ingredients:

Radix Codonopsis Pilosulae	12 g
Poria	9 g
Rhizoma Atractylodis Macrocephalae	9 g
Radix Glycyrrhizae	9 g
Semen Cassiae	9 g
Semen Celosiae	9 g
Aloe	9 g
Fructus Quisqualis	9 g
Fructus Crataegi	12 g
Massa Fermentata Medicinalis	12 g
Rhizoma Coptidis	6 g
Rhizoma Taraxaci	18 g

Administration: Decoct the above drugs in water for oral dose, once a day.

(3) Type of insufficiency of the spleen and stomach.

Symptoms and Signs: There is corneal ulceration or perforation, pale complexion, frequent diarrhoea and cool extremities.

Therepeutic Method: Warming the middle *Jiao*, dispelling cold and reinforcing the spleen and stomach.

Recipe: Modified *Fuzhi Lizhong Tang* (50)

Ingredients:

Radix Ginseng	9 g
Rhizoma Atractylodis Macrocephalae	9 g
Rhizoma Dioscoreae	9 g
Radix Aconiti Praeparata	9 g
Rhizoma Zingiberis	9 g
Radix Rehmanniae Praeparata	15 g
Radix Astragali seu Hedysari	15 g
Radix Paeoniae Alba	15 g
Pericarpium Citri Reticulatae	12 g
Flos Chrysanthemi	12 g

Administration: Decoct the above drugs in water for oral dose, once a day.

2. Other Therapies

(1) For local medication please refer to 9.1 corneal ulcer.

(2) Vitamins A and D for oral intake or for injection.

(3) Acupuncture Treatment: Needle any 3 or 4 of the points: Zhongwan, Zusanli, Weiyu, Piyu, Ganyu, etc. Once a day.

(4) Massage therapy may be used to recuperate the function of the spleen and the stomach.

(5) Propietary: *Renshen Jianpi Wan* (104) or *Shiquan Dabu Wan* (105)

For oral administration, 9 g. each time, twice daily.

10 Uveal Diseases

The uvea, containing an abundance of vessels, is sensitive to invasion of certain allergens or to affection of some general or local inflammatory diseases and hence the etiology is very complex. Uveitis may damage the visual function seriously, especialy the chonic ones which may finally result in blindness and atrophy of the globe due to the occurence of complications. Uveal diseases refer to disorder of the pupil in ophthalmology of TCM. The pupil means water orbiculus in terms of five orbiculi, corresponding to the kidney. Because the liver and the kidney have a common source, differention of types should be made mainly in consideration of the liver and the kidney. The etiology may be dysfunction of *Zang-Fu* organs or affection by exogenous pathogens. Therefore the focus should be detected before treatment based on type differentiation is given and the treatment should be aimed at the focus.

10.1 Acute Exudative Iridocyclitis

The disease mainly afflicts the anterior uveal. If the inflammation attacks repeatedly or the condition is serious, it may spread to the posterior uveal and develop into pan-uveitis, which is called *Tongshen Jinxiao* in TCM.

Etiology and Pathogenesis

It is usually due to the attack of wind-heat of the liver channel on the eye, or due to accumulation and steaming of dampness-heat which attacks the seven orifices and burns the pupils. Involvement by other diseases of the eye may also cause the disease.

Clinical Manifestations

Acute onset, pain in the eye, photophobia, lacrimation and blurred vision. Examinations may reveal ciliary congestion or mixed congestion. There exists tenderness in the ciliary region, greyish-white or pigment-like exudate attached to the lower part of the corneal endothelium, the congestion and swelling of the iris with indistinct markings, and aqueous opacity. In severe cases, the anterior chamber may present fibrinous exudate with colloid aqueous. There is such symptoms as miosis, retardation or loss of photoreaction and hypopsia.

Type and Treatment

1. Internal treatment

(1) Type of wind-heat of the liver channel.

Symptoms and Signs: There is acute onset, ophthalmalgia, photophobia, blacrimation, blurred vision, ciliary congestion, aqueous opacity, contracted pupil, accompanied with headache, thirst with dry throat, reddened tongue with thin and yellowish fur, and floating, rapid pulse.

Therapeutic Method: Dispelling wind and removing heat.

Recipe: Modified *Xinzhi Chailian Tang* (39)

Ingredients:

Radix Bupleuri	9 g
Rhizoma Coptidis	9 g
Radix Scutellariae	9 g
Fructus Gardeniae	9 g
Radix Gentianae	9 g

Caulis Akebiae	9 g
Herba Schizonepetae	9 g
Radix Ledebouriellae	9 g
Radix Paeoniae Rubra	12 g
Fructus Viticis	12 g
Cortex Mori Radicis	12 g
Radix Glycyrrhizae	6 g

Administration: Decoct the above drugs in water for oral dose, once a day.

(2) Type of retention of dampness−heat in the body.

Symptoms and Signs: The eye symptoms are exacerbated, There is mixed congestion, aqueous apacity, fibrinous exudates in the anterior chamber, bitter taste, dry throat, reddened tongue with yellowish and greasy fur, wiry and smooth pulse.

Therapeutic Method: Clearing away heat and promoting diuresis.

Recipe: Modified *Yiyang Jiulian San* (51)

Ingredients:

Radix Angelicae Pubescentis	9 g
Rhizoma seu Radix Notopterygii	9 g
Radix Stephaniae Tetrandrae	9 g
Radix Angelicae Dahuricae	9 g
Radix Ledebouriellae	9 g
Fructus Viticis	9 g
Radix Scutellariae	9 g
Rhizoma Coptidis	9 g
Fructus Gardeniae	9 g
Cortex Phellodendri	9 g
Rhizoma Anemarrhenae	9 g

   Radix Glycyrrhizae   9 g
   Radix Rehmanniae   15 g

Administration: Decoct the above drugs in water for oral dose, once a day.

2. Other Therapies

(1) Apply mydriatic to the eye so as to avoid posterior synechia and relieve the pain.

(2) Damp and hot compresses, half an hour a time, three times daily.

(3) Acupuncture treatment. The most commonly used acupoints are Jingming. Taiyang. Sibai, Sizhukong, Hegu, Zusanli, etc. Needle three local points and two distal points each time, once daily.

10.2 Chronic Uveitis

The disease is a chronic inflammation of the entire uveal tract, which usually develops from the acute inflammation. It corresponds to *Tongshen Ganque* in TCM.

Etiology and Patholgenesis

It is usually due to hyperactivity and flaming up of asthenic fire, a result of *Yin* —deficiency caused by long—term illness. or it may also be due to *Yang* —deficiency of the spleen and the kidney and decline of fire at the gate of life, which leads to the poor nourishment of channels and vessels.

Clinical Manifestations

In mild cases, there is no uncomfortable signs but the vision is gradually reduced. Examinations may detect slight ciliary congestion, a small amount of deposits in the posterior wall of the cornea, slight aqueous opacity, indistinct markings of the iris, depigmentation of the pupillary margin, posterior synechiae, or in some cases, Koeppe's nodules, coremetamorphosis, dust-like or flocculent opacities of the vitreous. In cases with protracted course, there is circular posterior synechiae, periipheral anterior synechia, synechia of the anterior chamber angle resulting in the rise of intraocular pressure. The patient may feel distention of the eye, headache, marked diminution of vision. The disease may also result in loss of vision because of the concurrent lenticular turbidity. If chronic inflammation is not controlled, it will finally cause atrophy of the eyeball and complete blindness.

Type and Treatment

1. Internal Treatment

(1) Type of hyperactivity of fire due to *Yin* deficiency.

Symptoms and Signs: Mild illness, chronic course, and repeated recurrence at times, accompanied with sleeplessness due to vexation, dysphoria with feverish sensation in chest, palms and sores, dry tongue and throat, reddened tongue with little coating, and small, rapid pulse.

Therapeutic Method: Nourishing *Yin* and reducing pathogenic fire.

Recipe: Modified *Zhibai Dihuang Tang* (43)

Ingredients:

Rhizoma Anemarrhenae	9 g
Cortex Phellodendri	9 g
Cortex Moutan Radicis	9 g
Rhizoma Alismatis	9 g
Poria	9 g
Radix Rehmanniae	15 g
Radix Scrophulariae	15 g

Radix Ophiopogonis	15 g
Radix Paeoniae Rubra	15 g
Radix Glycyrrhizae	6 g

Administration: Decoct the above drugs in water for oral dose, once a day.

(2) Type of *Yang* —dificiency of both the spleen and kidney.

Symptoms and Signs: Precence of all the symptoms of chronic uveitis, accompanied with aversion to cold, watery saliva, pale tongue with white fur, and sunken pulse.

Therapeutic Method: Warming and tonifying the spleen and kidney.

Recipe: Modified *Fuzi Lizhong Tang* (50)

Ingredients:

Radix Aconiti Praeparata	9 g
Rhizoma Atraclylodis Macrocephalae	9 g
Rhizoma Zingiberis	9 g
Praeparata Fructus Gardeniae	9 g
Radix Scutellariae	9 g
Radix Codonopsis Pilosulae	15 g
Radix Astragali seu Hedysari	15 g
Radix Paeoniae Alba	15 g
Radix Glycyrrhizae Praeparata	9 g

Administration: Decoct the above drugs in water for oral dose, once a day.

2. Other Therapies

(1) Regional medication is the same as for acute exudative iridocyclitis.

(2) Surgical operation should be considered if there is secondary glaucoma, complicated cataract.

(3) Propietary: *Mingmu Dihuang Wan* (114), or, *Shihu Yeguang Wan* (109), for oral administration 9 g a time, twice a day.

11 Diseases of the Lens

Diseases of the lens may be classified into 3 major types: (1) congenital anomalies of the lens; (2) dislocation of the lens; (3) lens opacity. If there is opacity in any part of the cortex, nucleus and capsule of the lens, it is termed a cataract. It may be classified into two types: the congenitial and the acquired. Here we will deal with senile cataract and traumatic cataract that TCM tharapies can treat with very good effects.

11.1 Senile Cataract

Senile cataract is one of the most common of acquired cataracts which is a manifestation of senile degeneration. In TCM, it belongs to the category of round cataract.

Etiology and Pathogenesis

In most instances senile debility with consequent deficiency of the liver and kidney, insufficiency of essence and blood, scarcity of *Qi* and blood, often leads to malnutrition of the eyes and causes the disease; Apart from this, dysfunction of the spleen in transportation of essence and energy for nourishment of the eyes may also be a cause to produce the disease.

Clinical Manifestations

At the early stage, the patient complains of black shadows occupying a fixed position in the visual field. Usually, monocular diplopia, polyopia or refraction change may occur. The occurance of visual disturbance depends upon the position which the opacities occupied in the lens.

1. Cortical cataract is most common seen. Clinicaly, the course consists of four stages.

Incipient stage: The lens under the pupil is transparent and after mydriasis, wedged opacities can be seen on the equator of the lens. In this stage, the condition develops slowly and has no interference with vision.

Immature stage (the stage of swelling): the wedged opacities on the equator gradually involve the pupillary zone and get deeper. The anterior chamber is reduced in depth. The examination by oblique illumination shows that the iris casts a semi–lunar shadow on the other side when the eye is illuminated from one side. There is obvious diminution of vision. During this stage, the lens swells. For a patient with glaucoma diathesis, the disease may induce glaucoma.

Mature stage: The cortex of the lens presents grayish–white panopacity. The shadow cast by the iris has disappeared. The anterior chamber regains its normal depth. There is mere perception of light.

Hypermature stage: The cataract has been mature for too long a period and the cloudy cortex may present milky liquefaction, calcification or deposits of cholesterin. The nucleus sinks to the bottom of this fluid. The upper part of the anterior chamber may become deeper. The iris may become tremulous.

2. Senile nuclear cataract is less common seen. The lens may present brown or amber opacity. When the lens turns black, it is known as black cataract. The cortex may still be transparent, but vision falls markedly. The disease progresses slowly. The opacity in the cortex may not occur for several years.

Type and Treatment

The course of the disease is fairly long. Medication may be effective in the incipient stage. When there is notable opacity of the lens, medicine will not work, and so surgical treatment should be considered.

1. Internal Treatment

(1) Type of deficiency of the liver and kidney.

Symptoms and Signs: Senile debility, blurred vision, dizziness and tinnitus, sorenese in loins and knees, pale tongue, and small, weak pulse.

Therapeutic Method: Tonifying the liver and kidney.

Recipe: Modified *Qiju Dihuang Tang* (52)

Ingredients:

Rhizoma Rehmanniae Praeparatae	24 g
Fructus Corni	12 g
Rhizoma Dioscoreae	12 g
Rhizoma Alismatis	9 g
Poria	9 g
Cortex Moutan Radicis	9 g
Fructus Lycii	9 g
Flos Chrysanthemi	9 g

Administration: Decoct the above drugs in water for oral dose, once daily.

(2) Type of Insufficiency of Spleen−*Qi*.

Symptoms and Signs: Blurred vision, listlessness, lassitude of the extremities, sallow complexion, poor appetite and loose stools, pale tongue with white fur, and slow or small weak pulse.

Therapeutic Method: Invigorating the spleen and replenishing *Qi*.

Recipe: Modified *Yiqi Congming Tang* (53)

Ingredients:

Fructus Viticis	12 g
Radix Astragali seu Hedysari	6 g
Radix Ginseng	6 g
Cortex Rhellodendri	9 g
Radix Paeoniae	9 g
Radix Glycyrrhizae Praeparata	3 g
Radix Puerariae	3 g

Administration: Decoct the above drugs in water for oral dose, once a day.

(3) Type of deficiency of *Yin* accompanied by dampness and heat.

Symptoms and Signs: Blurred vision, foreign body sensation in the eye, dysphoria with smothery sensation and halitosis, thirst but having no desire for drink, dry stools, and reddened tongue with yellowish fur.

Therapeutic Method: Nourishing *Yin,* clearing away heat, regulating *Qi* of the middle–*Jiao* and removing dampness by diuresis.

Recipe: Modified *Ganlu Yin* (54)

Ingredients:

Radix Rehmanniae	9 g
Rhizoma Rehmanniae Praeparatae	9 g
Herba Dendrobii	9 g
Radix Asparagi	12 g
Radix Ophiopogonis	12 g
Radix Scutellariae	9 g
Herba Artemisiae Scopariae	9 g

Radix Glycyrrhizae	6 g
Folium Eriobotryae	24 g

Administration: Decoct the above drugs in water for oral dose, once a day.

2. Other Therapies

(1) Propietary: *Shihu Yeguang Wan* (109) can be orally used for cases with deficiency of the liver and kidney. 9 g. each time, three times a day.

Buzhong Yiqi Wan (115) can be used for cases with insufficiency of spleen−*Qi*. 18 g. each time, twice a day.

(2) Acupuncture Treatment: This treatment is prescribed for patients at the incipient stage and it is better to be supported with medicines for oral administration. The commonly used acupoints are Jingming, Qiuhou, Zuanzhu, Yuyao, Binao, Hegu, Zusanli and Sanyinjiao. Needling is done once everyday or every other day at 2−3 points, 8−10 times as a cure.

(3) Eye droppings of Phacolysin, Catalin, 3 times a day.

(4) Surgical Treatment: If the above therapies do not work, the patient should wait until the mature stage for surgical treatment.

11.2 Traumatic Cataract

Traumatic cataract may result from a dull contusion or perforated wound. It is put into the category of *Jinzhen Neizhang* in TCM.

Etiology and Pathogenesis

The disease is mostly due to injuries to the blood vessels of the eyes, because they will lead to retention of blood stasis, dysfunction of *Qi* in controlling blood flow and stagnation of *Qi* and blood in the vessels, a condition that will gradually form cataract. Besides, stagnation of *Qi* and blood may cause obstruction of blood vessels and hinders refined substances from being sent upward to nourish the eyes, thus leading to everworsening blurred vision and finally to cataract.

Clinical Manifestations

In the cases of cataract caused by contusion, a small brownish ring-shaped opacity of pigment may be seen on the anterior capsule of the lens, which may subside spontaneously in several weeks or months, leaving a small spot of opacity or may be absorbed completely with no hinderance to vision. Sometimes, the cortex may present stellate, dendritic or coronary opacity, which usually develops slowly.

In the cases of cataract resulting from a penetrating wound, an opening on the capsule could be detected. Occasionally, the opacity of the lens remains limited to the injured portion after closure of the capsular opening and the opacity may cease to develop because the wound is small. If the opening is large, the opacity may involve the entire lens due to immersion of the aqueous humor. If the turbid cortex protrudes into the anterior chamber, secondary uveitis or glaucoma may occur.

Type and Treatment

1. Internal Treatment

(1) Type of stagnancy of *Qi* and blood.

Symptoms and Signs: There is swelling and blood stasis in the eyelid of the injured eye, accompanied by ophthalmalgia and headache, platycoria, torpor photoreaction. In severe cases, hyphema may occur. The lens becomes slightly cloudy and finally all opaque after a sufficiently long period of time.

Therapeutic Method: Regulating the blood flow, removing stagnancy, expelling wind and alleviating pain.

Recipe: Modified *Chufeng Yisun Tang* (55)

Ingredients:

Rhizoma Angelicae Sinensis	6 g
Radix Paeoniae Alba	6 g
Rhizoma Rehmanniae Praeparata	6 g
Rhizoma Ligustici Chuanxiong	6 g
Rhizoma Ligustici	5 g
Radix Peucedani	5 g
Radix Ledebouriellae	5 g
Cortex Moutan Radicis	9 g
Radix Notoginseng	3 g
Flos Carthami	6 g

Administration: Decoct the above drugs in water for oral dose, once a day.

(2) Type of deficiency of the liver and kidney.

Symptoms and Signs: In late stage of the disease, the eyes are neither red nor swelling despite of existence of part of the cataract.

Therapeutic Method: Tonifying the liver and kidney.

Recipe: Modified *Mingmu Dihuang Tang* (56)

Ingredients:

Rhizoma Rehmanniae Preaparata	24 g
Fructus Corni	12 g
Rhizoma Dioscoreae	12 g
Rhizoma Alismatis	9 g
Poria cum Ligno Hospite	9 g
Cortex Moutan Radicis	9 g

Radix Rehmanniae	24 g
Radix Bupleuri	12 g
Radix Angelicae Sinensis	12 g
Fructus Schisandrae	9 g

Administration: Decoct the above drugs in water for oral dose, once a day.

2. Other Therapies

(1) Proprietary: *Mingmu Dihuang Wan* (114) can be orally used for cases at the late stage when the cataract begins to take form, 18 g. each time, twice a day.

(2) If medication fails to work due to long-term opacity but the patient still has light and color perceptions, surgical treatment can be applied in half a year. If secondary glaucoma occurs, it had better be managed with surgical treatment as timely as possible.

12 Glaucoma

Glaucoma is an ocular disease caused by increase of intraocular pressure leading to the injury of the visual function. It is classified into three categories. They are primary glaucoma, congenital glaucoma and secondary glaucoma. The first two categories involve both eyes while the secondary one occurs mainly in one eye. Primary glaucoma is further divided into open-angle type and angel closure type. In TCM, glaucoma corresponds to *Wufeng Neizhang* included in disorders of the pupil, that is, *Lufeng Neizhang, Qingfeng Neizhang, Wufeng Neizhang, Heifeng Neizhang* and *Huangfeng Neizhang*. Among them, *Lufeng Neizhang* and *Qingfeng Neizhang* are more commonly seen in clinical practice and will be dealt with in this part.

12.1 Acute Angle Closure Glaucoma

Acute angle closure glaucoma, usually found in old females, involves both eyes, but at first it may just affect one eye. The interval between the occurrences of syndromes of the two eyes is irregular. The attack is usually caused by mental depression or overwork. The onset is acute with the characteristics of sudden distention, conjunctival congestion, sudden diminution of vision, accompanied by nausea and vomiting. It is termed *Lufeng Neizhang* in TCM.

Etiology and Pathogenesis

The disease is due to long-standing stagnation of the liver *Qi* caused by emotional upset, which later turns into fire to attack the eyes; it may also be due to flaming of fire of the liver and gallbladder which may develop into wind-heat to attack the eyes, or due to retention of phlegmdampness that turns into fire to attack the eyes. Besides, damage of *Yin* caused by overstain may lead to hyperactivity of *Yang* and induce endogenous wind. When the wind goes upward to attack the eyes, the disease occurs.

Clinical Manifestations

There are four stages according to the progress of pathogeny. At the preclinical stage, following an emotional stress, there is mild headache, distention in the eye and iridization but the symptoms may have spontaneous remission after rest. At the stage of attack, there is distending pain in the eyeball, severe headache, nausea, vomiting and sudden diminution of vision due to rapid increase of the intraocular pressure. An examination may reveal mixed congestion, corneal edema which presents ground-glass-like opacity, a shallow anterior chamber, fan-shaped iridoatrophy, mydriasis, disappearance of photoreaction, and grayish-white cloudy spots under the anterior capsule of the lens. The anterior chamber angles are closed. At the remission stage, the intraocular pressure reduces as a result of treatment, the symptoms subside; the visual function improves; congestion disappears; the cornea clears up; and the anterior chamber angle reopens. But if high intraocular pressure persists, the anterior chamber may become adherent. The duration of this stage varies. At the chronic stage, an acute attack that has not yet been timely treated, or repeated attacks, would lead to extensive adhesion of the anterior chamber angles, which results in continuous increase of the intraocular pressure, marked diminution of vision, contraction of visual field, higher ratio between the cup and the optic disc and pale color of the disc. The blood vessels are pushed to the nasal side, like bending-knees. The chamber angle becomes narrower or closed. Gradually the vision will completely lose and the disease will enter the absolute stage.

Type and Treatment

1. Internal Treatment

(1) Type of stagnation of the liver—Qi.

Symptoms and Signs: Congestion and distending pain of the eye, iridization, diminution of vision, emotional upset, headache, chest distress, nausea, vomiting, reddened tongue with thin fur, and wiry, small pulse.

Therapeutic Method: Relieving the depressed liver. Removing heat and expelling wind.

Recipe: Modified *Danzhi Xiaoyao San* (57)

Ingredients:

Radix Bupleuri	9 g
Cortex Moutan Radicis	9 g
Fructus Cardeniae	9 g
Rhizoma Atractylodis Macrocephalae	9 g
Poria	9 g
Radix Glycyrrhizae	9 g
Radix Paeoniae Alba	12 g
Radix Angelicae Sinensis	12 g
Rhizoma Pinelliae	12 g
Radix Angelicae Dahuricae	12 g
Flos Chrysanthemi	12 g
Fired Semen Ziziphi	30 g

Administration: Decoct the above drugs in water for oral dose, once a day.

(2) Type of flaming of fire in the liver and gallbladder.

Symptoms and Signs: There are all the symptoms of the angle closure glaucoma, accompanied with nausea, vomiting, aversion to cold, fever, deep-colored urine, constipation, reddened tongue with yellow fur, and wiry, rapid pulse.

Therapeutic Method: Purging the liver of pathogenic fire.

Recipe: Modified *Lufeng Lingyang Yin* (58)

Ingredients:

Radix Scutellariae	9 g
Rhizoma Anemarrhenae	9 g
Radix et Rhizoma Rhei	9 g
Radix Ledebouriellae	9 g
Rhizoma Alismatis	9 g
Spica Prunellae	9 g
Radix Scorphulariae	12 g
Poria	12 g
Semen Plantaginis	12 g
Pulvis Corun Autelopis	3 g

(Taking it after its infusion with the decoction)

Administration: Decoct the above drugs in water for oral dose, once a day.

(3) Type of upward disturbance of phlegm-fire.

Symptoms and Signs: Conjunctival congestion, distending pain of the eye, blurred vision, headache, nausea, vomiting, dizziness, deep-colored urine, constipation reddened tongue with yellow and greasy fur, and smooth, rapid pulse.

Therapeutic Method: Removing heat and expelling phlegm.

Recipe: Modified *Banxia Lingyangjiao San* (59)

Ingredients:

Corun Saigae Tataricae	9 g
Herba Menthae	9 g
Rhizoma seu Radix Notopterygii	9 g
Radix Ledebouriellae	9 g
Rhizoma Pinelliae	9 g
Rhizoma Ligustis Chuanxiong	9 g
Rhizoma Alismatis	9 g
Pericarpium Citri Reticulatae	9 g
Fructus Viticis	12 g
Flos Chrysanthemi	12 g
Semen Cassiae	12 g
Semen Plantaginis	15 g

Administration: Decoct the above drugs in water for oral dose, once a day.

(4) Type of hyperactivity of *Yang* due to *Yin* deficiency.

Symptoms and Signs: There is a feeling of dullness and a slight pain in the eye and the head, blurred vision, dysphoria and irritation, tinnitus, deafness, dry mouth and throat, reddened tongue with little coating, and small, rapid pulse.

Therapeutic Method: Nourishing *Yin* and clearing away heat.

Recipe: Modified *Lingyang Gouteng Yin* (60)
Ingredients:

Ramulus Uncariae cum Uncis	12 g
Folium Mori	12 g
Flos Chrysanthemi	12 g
Poria	12 g
Radix Rehmanniae	15 g
Radix Paeoniae Alba	15 g

Rhizoma Pinelliae	9 g
Caulis Bambusae in Taeniam	9 g
Radix Glycyrrhizae	9 g
Pulvis Corun Saigae Tataricae	3 g

(Taking it after its infusion with the decoction.)

Administration: Decoct the above drugs in water for oral dose.

2. Other Therapies

(1) 2% Semen Arecae Fluid (110), or 1% Caulis Erycibes Fluid (101) can be used to instil eyes, three times daily.

(2) Acupuncture Treatment: The commonly used points are Jingming, Sibai, Chengqi, Qiuhou, Hegu, Taichong and Fengchi, Choose four points for needling, once a day.

(3) Auriculo-acupuncture: Search for sensitive points and use them in coordination with the points eye 1, eye 2, liver, etc. for needle-embedding or Semen Vaccaria plaster mounting until the remission of the symptoms.

12.2 Open-angle Glaucoma

Open-angle glaucoma, which is also called Simple Glaucoma, is characterized by pathological increase of the intraocular pressure and an open anterior chamber angle. As it progresses slowly with slight symptoms, it is not easy to detect it at the early stage. The disease is usually found in young adults, and males are affected more often than females. It corresponds to *Qingfeng Neizhang* in TCM.

Etiology and Pathogenesis

Emotional depression of a person may cause stagnation of the liver *Qi* that will turn into fire. When the fire goes upward to attack the eyes, the disease occurs. Or, if a person suffers from retention of dampness due to hyperfunction of the spleen, phlegm will originate from the retention and form phlegm stagnation which will further convert into fire. When the fire moves upward to attack the eye, the disease is caused. Besides, deficiency of the liver and kidney, a condition called consumption of primordal *Yin,* will result in asthenic fire, and attack of the eye by the fire will lead to the disease.

Clinical Manifestations

At the early stage there is almost no symptom, but slight distention feeling in the eyes, headache and iridization may occur due to overwork or emotional upset. As the disease progresses, vision diminishes and visual field shrinks gradually and blindness will occur finally. Clinical examination shows that there is no change in the anterior part of the eye. The cupping of the disc of the fundus becomes wider and deeper. The cupdisc ratio is above 0.5. The blood vessels are pushed to the nasal side, some of which look like bending knees, with nerve fiber layer defect. At the late stage the optic disc is pallor and look like a cup. The anterior chamber angle is wide. The intraocular pressure is elevated and its undulation amplitude is large within twenty-four hours.

Type and Treatment

1. Internal Treatment

(1) Type of fire due to stagnation of *Qi.*

Symptoms and Signs: Slight distention feeling in the eye, iridization, headache, dizziness, fullness in the chest and hypochondria, reddened tongue with yellow fur, and wiry, small pulse.

Therapeutic Method: Clearing away heat and relieving the

liver.

Recipe: Modified *Danzhi Xiaoyao San* (57)
Ingredients:

Radix Bupleuri	9 g
Cortex Moutan Radicis	9 g
Fructus Gardeniae	9 g
Poria	9 g
Rhizoma Atractylodis Macrocephalae	9 g
Radix Angeicae Dahuricae	9 g
Flos Chrysanthemi	9 g
Spica Drunellae	9 g
Radix Paeoniae Alba	12 g
Radix Angelicae sinensis	12 g
Ramulus Uncariae cum Uncis	12 g
Pulvis Cornu Saigae Tataricae	3 g

(Taking it after its infusion with the decoction.)

Administration: Decoct the above drugs in water for oral dose, once a day.

(2) Type of combined attack of fire and phlegm.

Symptoms and Signs: There are all the eye symptoms of open-angle glaucoma, accompanied with dizziness, bitter taste and dry throat, fullness in the chest and hypochondria, irritability, reddened tongue with yellow and greasy fur, and smooth, rapid pulse.

Therapeutic Method: Clearing away heat and removing phlegm.

Recipe: Modified *Lingyang Jiao San* (61)
Ingredients:

Pulvis Cornu Saigae Tataricae	3 g

Flos Chrysanthemi	12 g
Semen Cassiae	12 g
Fructus Viticis	12 g
Radix Ophiopogonis	12 g
Poria cum Ligno Hospite	12 g
Radix Paeoniae Rubra	12 g
Semen Plantaginis	12 g
Canlis Bambusae in Taeniam	9 g
Rhizoma Pinelliae	9 g
Arisaema cum Bile	9 g
Radix Glycyrrhizae	9 g

Administration: Decoct the above drugs in water for oral dose, once a day.

(3) Type of deficiency of the liver and kidney.

Symptoms and Signs: There are all the eye symptoms of open-angle glaucoma, together with insomnia, amnesia, soreness and weakness of loins and knees, dizziness, tinnitus, red tongue with little coating, small and rapid pulse.

Therapeutic Method: Nourishing the liver and kidney

Recipe: Modified *Qiju Dihuang Tang* (52)

Ingredients:

Fructus Lycii	12 g
Flos Chrysanthemi	12 g
Rhizoma Rehmanniae Praeparatae	12 g
Radix Paeoniae Alba	12 g
Radix Codonopsis Pilosulae	12 g
Poria cum Ligno Hospite	12 g
Rhizoma Alismatis	9 g
Seman Plantaginis	9 g

Rhizoma Gastrodiae　　　　　　　　　　　　9 g

Administration: Decoct the above drugs in water for oral dose, once a day.

2. Other Therapies

(1) Using 1% Canlis Erycibes Fluid to instil eyes, three times daily.

(2) Using 2% Semen Arecae Fluid to instil eyes, three times daily.

(3) Using the same accupuncture treatment as for acute angle closure glaucoma.

13 Diseases of the Optic Fundus

Diseases of the optic fundus are quite numerous; TCM therapies can produce very good results in treating some of them and we just discuss these ones in this chapter.

13.1 Obstruction of the Central Retinal Vessels

Obstruction of the central retinal vessels includes occlusion of the central retinal artery and thrombosis of central retinal vein. The visual acuity drops rapidly in the former and slowly in the latter. In some cases, secondary glaucoma may happen. The disease is put into the category of *Baomang* in TCM.

Etiology and Pathogenesis

A person's violent rage is often followed by hyperactivity of liver—*Qi* that tends to cause stagnation of *Qi* and blood. When the stagnation forms obstruction of the vessels in the retina, the disease occurs. Intemperance in drinking and indulgence in taking pungent foods may also lead to the disease because this habit will result in retention of stomach—heat and dysfunction of *Ying—Qi* (the nutritive system). If the dysfuction causes obstruction of blood flow in the retina, the disease may follow. Other causes of the disease may be overstrain of the mind or eyes, or uncontrolled sexual life. In any of these cases, the result will be consumption of primordial *Yin* without the person's knowing it, thus giving rise to hyperactive liver—*Yang*, When the liver *Yang* goes up to attack the upper orifices, especially the eyes, the disease takes place. In addition, dysfunction of the spleen in transportation will cause stagnation and accumulation of dampness and phlegm in association with disharmmony between *Qi* and blood, and this may induce ascension of *Yang* and agitation of endogenous wind. If the wind combines with the phlegm, they will form obstruction to the channels. Hence the disease occurs.

Clinical Manifestations

The disease usually has a sudden onset, with abrupt and complete anopia or rapid hyposia in a few days. But there is no external signs. Examination of the fundus: In cases of occlusion of the central retinal artery, the retina shows anemia and the part of it at the posterior polar becomes grayish white, milky, edematous. There is a cherry—red spot in the region of the macula. The optic papilla becomes white with blurred margins. There is no pulsation of the artery when the eyeball is pressed. The arteries of the retina become very thin giving a white thread appearance. In cases with thrombosis of the central retinal vein, the optic papilla shows obvious hyperemia, and edema with indistinct margins. The retina shows edema and the veins are enormously distended and very tortuous in purplish red color. Sometimes the vein may hide in the edematous retina or be mixed with the blood spots presenting a segmental apprearance. The artery becomes thinner. There are a large amount of superficial flame—shaped, radial and deep round—shaped blood spots and cotten—wool exudate in the retina and optic papilla. When there is large amount of hemorrhage, the blood may get into the vitreous. If this condition lasts long, on the surface of the optic papilla and the surroundings of the affected veins, new capillary—net may grow and secondary glaucoma may develop.

Type and Treatment

These two types of syndrome discribed above may severely impair the vision. So attention must be paid to them. Clinically, emergency treatment of both TCM and Western medicine should be given promptly in accordance with the etiology. Then normal treatment of the disease can begin according to the condition of the patient, the course of the disease and general differentiation of symptoms and signs.

1. Internal Treatment

(1) Type of stagnation of *Qi* and blood.

Symptoms and Signs: There is sudden loss of vision during the onset and all the changes mentioned above such as dizziness, headache, distension and pain in the chest and hypochondria and taut pulse or taut, uneven pulse may accur.

Therapeutic Method: Promoting blood circulation and removing obstruction from the orifices

Recipe: Modified *Tongqiao Huoxue Tang* (62)

Ingredients:

Radix Paeoniae Rubra	3 g
Rhizoma Ligustici Chuanxiong	3 g
Semen Persicae (Mashed)	9 g
Flos Carthami	9 g
Allium Fistulosum	3 g
Fructus Ziziphi Jujubae	7 pieces
Moschus	1.5 g
(Be decoted later)	
Radix Curaumae	9 g
Pericarpium Citri Reticulatae Viride	6 g

Administration: Decoct the above drugs in water for oral

dose, 1 dosage daily, which is taken before going to bed at night.

Modifications: 1. For cases with severe edema of the retina, add:

Succinum	6 g
Herba Lycopi	9 g
Herba Leonuri	12 g

2. For cases with copious hemorrhage in the eyeground add:

Pollen Typhae	12 g
Radix Rubiae	12 g
Radix Notoginseng	6 g

(2) Type of excessiveness of phlegm and heat.

Symptoms and Signs: The patient may have the same eye symptoms as those of the last type. Meanwhile, the patient may feel vertigo and heaviness in the head, oppressed feeling in the chest, dysphoria, poor appetite, nausea, thick phlegm and bitter taste, yellow and greasy coating, and taut, slippery pulse.

Therapeutic Method: Romoving phlegm and relieving the obstruction of orifices.

Recipe: Modified *Di Tan Tang* (63)

Ingredients:

Rhizoma Pinelliae	8 g (Praeparata)
Arisaema cum Bile	8 g
Exocarpium Citri Grandis	
Fructus Aurantii Immaturus	6 g
Poria	6 g
Radix Ginseng	3 g
Acorus Calamus	3 g
Caulis Bambusaw in Taeniam	2 g

Radix Glycyrrhizae	2 g
Rhizoma Zingiberis Recens	6 g
Fructus Ziziphi Jujubae	7 pieces
Bombyx Batryticatus	6 g
Lumbricus	12 g
Rhizoma Ligustici Chuanxiong	8 g

Administration: Decoct the above drugs in water for oral dose, one dose daily.

(3) Type of up-stirring of liver-wind.

Eye symptoms are the same as those described above in (1) The general symptoms are dizziness, tinnitus, flushed face, dysphoria, irritability, insomia, reddened tongue, yellow coating, taut pulse and in some cases lassitude in loins and knees, nocturnal emission and weariness, scarlet tongue and thready pulse.

Therapeutic Methods: Calming the liver, nourishing *Yin* and eliminiating the wind.

Recipe: Modified *Tianma Gouteng Yin* (64)

Ingredients:

Rhizoma Gastrodiae	9 g
Ramulus Uncariae cum Uncis	12 g
(To be decocted later)	
Concha Haliotidis	18 g
(Be decocted ahead of the other medicines)	
Fructus Gardeniae	9 g
Radix Scutellariae	9 g
Radix Cyathulae	12 g
Cortex Eucommiae	9 g
Herba Leonuri	9 g
Ramulus Loranthi	9 g

Caulis Polygoni Multiflori	12 g
Poria cum Ligno Hospite Rubra	9 g
Radix Paeoniae	12 g
Colla Corii Asini	6 g
Radix Salviae Miltiorrhizae	15 g
Lumbricus	12 g

Administration: Decoct the above drugs in water for oral dose, one dose daily.

2. Other Therapies

(1) Propietary: *Qiju Dihuang Wan* (110) for oral administration at the late stage of the disease. 18 g a time, twice a day.

(2) For the cases with emobolism of the central retinal artery, vasodilator should be given promptly for emergency management, such as Isoamyl nitrite as an inhalant or nitroglycerin as a perlingual cure used sublingually.

(3) Acupuncture Treatment: The periorbital points commonly used are Jingming, Qiuhou, Tongziliao, Chengqi, Zuanzhu, Taiyang. The distal points are Fengchi, Hegu, Neiguan, Waiguan, Taichong, Yifeng, Zuguangming, Mingmen, Shenshu. Choose 2 periorbital points and 2 distal points in turn every day. Give acupuncture only, do not retain the needle nor apply any moxibustion.

13.2 Retinal Periphlebitis

The disease is characterized with retinal hemorrhage and changes of retinal veins. It often occurs in young males of 21–30 years old and usually affects the eyes one after the other. It is apt to occur repeatedly. In TCM, it falls into *Yunwu Yijing* or *Baomang*.

Etiology and Pathogenesis

The disease is usually due to extravasation which results from the injury of *Ying* system by endogenous fire—heat, or due to derangement of *Qi* and blood which results from stagnancy of deficient fire in the vessels caused by insufficiency of the liver and kidney. Apart from these, deficiency of *Qi* and bood in the heart and spleen may also lead to abnormal flood of *Qi* and blood, thus causing extravasation.

Clinical Manifestations

At the beginning of the disease, there is no obvious change of vision. But sometimes a few black shadows float up and down in the vision. Diminution of vision may suddenly occur because of changes of the patient's condition. The fundus presents very tortuous and enormously distended distal veins with white sheaths, and grayish white exudate and hemorrhage around the them. Slight bleeding may occur in the vitreous. If the bleeding is profuse, vitreous hyperopacity may occur. Profuse and repeated bleeding may cause hyperplasia of the connective tissues resulting in proliferating retinitis.

Type and Treatment

1. Internal Treatment

(1) Type of the attack of fire and heat leading to extravasation of blood.

Symptoms and Signs: Visual acuity drops suddenly. The veins of the optic fundus are congested and enormously distended. The bleeding is profuse in bright red color or there is vitreous homatocele and blurred optic fundus. The tongue is red with yellowish fur; the pulse condition is taut, thready and rapid.

Therapeutic Methods: Clearing away heat and purging fire,

removing heat from the blood and preventing bleeding

Recipe: Modified *Ning Xie Tang* (69)

Ingredients:

Herba Agrimoniae	12 g
Herba Ecliptae	12 g
Radix Rehmanniae	12 g
Fructus Gardeniae Carbonisetus	9 g
Radix Paeoniae	15 g
Radix Ampelopsis	9 g
Cacumen Biotae	9 g
Colla Corii Asini	6 g
Rhizoma Imperatae	15 g

Administration: Decoct the above drugs in water for oral dose, one dose daily.

Modifications: For cases with dysphoria and irritability, bitter taste and dry throat, add to the prescription:

Radix Gentianae	9 g
Spica Prunellae	12 g

(2) Type of hyperactivity of fire due to *Yin* deficiency, and impairment to the vessels by the fire.

Symptoms and Signs: There are repeated moderate bleedings which may be accompanied with some new-born vessels, reddened lips and flushed cheeks, bitter taste and dry throat, dizziness, tinnitus, lumbago, nocturnal emission, dysphoria with feverish sensation in the palms and soles, and scarlet tongue with little coating.

Therapeutic Method: Nourishing *Yin* and reducing pathogenic fire

Recipe: Modified *Zhibai Dihuang Tang* (43)

Ingredients:

Radix Rehmanniae Praeparatae	12 g
Fructus Corni	6 g
Rhizoma Dioscoreae	6 g
Rhizoma Alismatis	4.5 g
Poria	4.5 g
Cortex Moutan Radicis	4.5 g
Rhizoma Anemarrhenae	30 g
Cortex Phellodendri	30 g

Administration: Decoct the above durgs in water for oral dose, one dose daily.

(3) Type of deficiency of *Qi* and blood in the heart and spleen.

Symptoms and Signs: The blood spots in the fundus are palish red in color. The patient shows sallow complexion, lassitude, palpitation, anorexia, with poor appetite, loose stools, pale tongue and feeble pulse.

Therapeutic Method: Nourishing the heart and invigorating the spleen, supplementing *Qi* and improving eyesight.

Recipe: Modified *Gui Pi Tang* (82)

Ingredients:

Rhizoma Atractylodis Macrocephalae	30 g
Poria cum Ligno Hospite	30 g
Radix Astragali seu Hedysari	30 g
Arillus Longan	30 g
Semen Ziziphi Spionsae	30 g
Radix Ginseng	15 g
Radix Aucklandiae	15 g
Radix Glycyrrhizae Praeparata	8 g

Radix Angelicae Sinensis	3 g
Radix Polygalae	3 g (Praeparata)
Rhizoma Zingiberis Recens	6 g
Fructus Ziziphi Jujubae	7 pieces

Administration: Decoct the above drugs in water for oral dose, one dose daily.

(4) Type of stagnation and accumulation of blood stasis.

Symptoms and signs: The desease is obstinate. Visual acuity does not improve obviously after a long time of treatment. The ecchymosis in the fundus is dark red in color, and in some cases the connective tissue gets proliferated. The tongue is purplish dark or with ecchymosis.

Therapeutic Methods: Promoting blood circulation by removing blood stasis, softening and resolving hard mass.

Recipe: Modified *Qu Yu Tang* (70)

Ingredients:

Radix Rehmanniae	25 g
Herba Ecliptae	15 g
Herba Agrimoniae	12 g
Semen Persicae	9 g
Radix Paeoniae Rubra	9 g
Herba Lycopi	12 g
Radix Salviae Miltiorrhizae	15 g
Rhizoma Ligustici Chuanxiong	9 g
Radix Curcumae	12 g
Radix Angelicae Sinensis	9 g

Administration: Decoct the above drugs in water for oral dose, one dose daily.

2. Other therapies

(1) Adopt the ion-introduction therapy with the solution of Radix Notoginseng or Flos Carthami.

(2) If the bleeding of vitreous body is copious and the condition is not improved after 3-6 months treatment, vitreous replacement should be considered.

13.3 Central Serous Choroidal Retinopathy

The disease is characterized by edema in the fundus macula area and metamorphopsia and blurred vision. Middle-aged males are susceptible to the disease. Usually it attacks one eye. In a few cases, the eyes are affected one after the other. The disease tends to recur repeatedly and it is put into the category of *Shi Zhan Hun Miao* in TCM.

Etiology and Pathogenesis

The disease may be due to: (1) dysfunction of the spleen, resulting in its failure to transport the refined substances to the eyes; (2) accumulation of phlegm-dampness in middle-*Jiao* and retention of dampness-heat in the body which disturbs the seven orifices; (3) emotional depression and obstruction of sweat pores leading to stagnancy of *Qi* and blood; (4) deficiency of liver-*Yin* and kidney-*Yin* and consumption of essence and blood leading to poor nourishment of the eyes; (5) consumption of the heart nutriment and energ; (6) improper use of the eyes and exhaustion of *Qi* and blood resulting in lustreless and spiritless eyes.

Clinical Manifestations

In early stage, there is a shadow in front of the visial field followed by diminution of central vision. There is a fixed black shadow at the center of the visual area. Micropsia or metamorphopsia exists in association with allochromasia.

Fundus examination: The macular area shows greyish red or greyish white discoid edema with round or oval light reflecting rings at its margin. There is absence of the central foveolar reflex. Then, yellowish white punctate exudate or small patch of bleeding appears in the macular area. At the restoration stage, edema and exudate are gradually absorbed. The pigment left at the macular area is distributed in disorder. The central foveolar reflex recovers and vision gradually restores.

Fluorescent exudate can be seen in the macular edema area under examination of Fluorescein Fundus Angiography (FFA)

Type and Treatment

1. Internal Treatment

(1) Type of upward invasion by turbid pathogenic factors.

Symptoms and Signs: The patient complains of blurred vision and metamorphosia. Macular edema, yellowish—white exudate spots and disappearance of central foveolar reflex can be seen in the optic fundus. The course of the disease usually lasts several years and the patient often has a heavy feeling of the head, oppressed feeling in the chest with poor appetite and bitter taste, scanty and dark—colored urine, yellow and greasy fur, and soft rapid pulse.

Therapeutic Methods: Removing dampness by diuresis, clearing away heat and removing phlegm dampness.

Recipe: *San Ren Tang* (7)

Ingredients:

Semen Armeniacae Amarum	15 g
Talcum	18 g
Medulla Tetrapanacis	6 g
Semen Amomi Cardamomi	6 g

Herba Lophatheri	6 g
Cortex Magnoliae officinalis	6 g
Semen Coicis	18 g
Rhizoma Pinelliae	6 g

Administration: Decoct the above drugs in water for oral dose. One dose daily.

Modifications: For cases with obvious macular edema, add to the prescription:

Fructus Leonuri	12 g
Rhizoma Alismatis	9 g
Semen Plantaginis	12 g

For cases of planty of exudate add:

Caulis Bambusae in Taeniam	12 g
Arisaema cum Bile	6 g
Fructus Aurantii	6 g

(2) Type of stagnancy of *Qi* and blood stasis.

Symptoms and Signs: There are all the eye symptoms of the type discussed above, accompanied by depressed emotion, dizziness, hypochondriac pain, dry throat, bitter taste, and rapid, wiry pulse.

Therapeutic Methods: Removing heat, relieving the depressed liver, promoting flow of *Qi* and invigorating blood circulation.

Recipe: *Dan Zhi Xiaoyao San* (57)

Ingredients:

Radix Bupleuri	15 g
Radix Angelicae Sinensis	15 g
Radix Paeoniae Alba	15 g
Rhizoma Atractylodis Macrocephalae	15 g

Poria	15 g
Radix Glycyrrhizae	3 g
Rhizoma Zingiberis Recens	2 slices
Herba Menthae	3 g
Cortex Moutan Radicis	3 g
Fructus Gardeniae	3 g

Administration: Decoct the above drugs in water for oral dose. One dose daily.

(3) Type of deficiency of the liver and kidney.

Symptoms and Signs: Dryness and foreign body sensation of the eyes, blurred vision, mild edema in the macular area with slight pigmentation, accompanied with dizziness, tinnitus, insomnia, or dreamful sleeping, soreness in the loins and knees, pale tongue with little fur and thready pulse.

Therapeutic Methods: Tonifying the liver and kidney.

Recipe: Modified *Zhujing Wan* (65)

Ingredients:

Semen Cuscutae	12 g
Fructus Broussonetiae	12 g
Fructus Leonuri	9 g
Fructus Lycii	6 g
Semen Plantaginis	6 g
Fructus Chaenomelis	6 g
Calcitum	6 g
Pulivis Placenta Hominis	9 g
(Be taken after its infusion with the decoction)	
Pulivis Radix Notoginseng	1.5 g
(Be taken after its infusion with the decoction)	
Fructus Schisandrae	6 g

Administration: Decoct the above drugs in water for oral dose. One dose daily.

(4) Type of deficiency of the heart and spleen.

Symptoms and Signs: Slow recovery of visual acuity, mild fundus edema with minimal exudate that cannot easily subside. Other accompanied symptoms and signs include dim complexion, dizziness and palpitation, poor appetite, lassitude, pale tongue and weak pulse.

Therapeutic Methods: Nourishing the heart and strengthening the spleen; Enriching the blood and promoting its circulation.

Recipe: *Renshen Yangrong Tang* (66)

Ingredients:

Radix Paeoniae Alba	30 g
Radix Angelicae Sinensis	10 g
Pericarpium Citri Reticulatae	10 g
Radix Astragali seu Hedysari	10 g
Lignum Cinnamomi	10 g
Radix Ginseng	10 g
Rhizoma Atractylodis Macrocephalae	10 g
Radix Glycyrrhizae Praeparata	10 g
Rhizoma Rehmanniae Praeparata	9 g
Fructus Schisandrae	9 g
Poria	9 g
Radix Polygalae Praeparata	6 g
Rhizoma Zingiberis Recens	3 slices
Fructus Ziziphi Jujubae	2 pieces

Administration: Decoct the above drugs in water for oral dose. One dose daily.

2. Other therapies

Acupuncture and moxibustion: The most frequently used acupuncture points are Jingming, Qiuhou, Toulingqi, Taiyang, Fengchi, Yiming, Hegu, Yanglao, Guangming, Ganshu, Shenshu, Zusanli etc. Select 2 local points and two distal points for needling, once daily. 10 days is a course.

13.4 Pigmentary Degeneration of the Retina

Pigmentary degeneration of the retina is a chronic progressive disease involving both eyes. It has an obvious familial hereditary factor. It is usually seen in males and termed *Gaofeng Neizhang* in TCM.

Etiology and Pathogenesis

The disease may be caused by: (1) decline of fire at the gate of life due to deficiency of the natural endowment; (2) deficiency of liver—*Yin* and kidney—*Yin* resulting in insufficiency of essence and blood; (3) weakness of the spleen and stomach and failure of lucid *Yang* in rising. All of these conditions will affect blood circulation in the vessels, resulting in sluggishness of blood circulation and poor nourishment of the eyes.

Clinical Manifestations

Usually both eyes are affected and there is night blindness. Photopic vision is not affected at the early stage, but as time passes, it drops by degrees. Visual field is a ring—shaped scotoma at the initial stage. Gradually, the concentric contraction of the field of vision becomes tubular and finally results in blindness. High stricture of retinal arteries and veins is seen in the optic fundus. Optic papilla shows waxen yellow or yellowish white color and there is bone—cell—like pigmentation of retina. Cataract and glaucoma may occur at the late stage.

Type and Treatment

1. Internal Treatment

(1) Type of decline of the fire at the gate of life.

Symptoms and Signs: The eye symptoms are the same as those of the disease discussed above. Other manifestations are aversion to cold with cold limbs, lassitude in loins and knees, frequent urination at night, pale tongue, and weak, sunken pulse.

Therapeutic Methods: Warming and recuperating kidney–*Yang*.

Recipe: *Yougui Wan* (67)

Ingredients:

Rhizoma Rehmanniae Praeparatae	24 g
Rhizoma Dioscoreae	12 g
Fructus Corni	9 g
Fructus Lycii	12 g
Colla Cornus Cervi	12 g
Semen Cuscutae	12 g
Cortex Eucommiae	12 g
Radix Angelicae Sinensis	9 g
Cortex Cinnamomi	12 g
Radix Aconiti Praeparata	6 g

Administration: Decoct the above drugs in water for oral dose. One dose daily.

(2) Type of deficiency of liver and kidney.

Symptoms and Signs: In addition to the symptoms and signs of the type mentioned above, there are sensation of dryness and discomfort of the eyes, dizziness and tinnitus, insomnia or dreamful sleeping, reddened tongue with little fur, rapid and thready pulse.

Therapeutic Methods: Nourishing the liver and kidney.

Recipe: Modified *Mingmu Dihuang Tang* (56)

Ingredients:

Rhizoma Rehmanniae Praeparatae	24 g
Fructus Corni	12 g
Rhizoma Dioscoreae	12 g
Rhizoma Alismatis	9 g
Poria cum Ligno Hospite	9 g
Cortex Moutan Radicis	9 g
Radix Rehmanniae	24 g
Radix Bupleuri	9 g
Radix Angelicae Sinensis	9 g
Fructus Schisandrae	6 g
Radix Salviae Miltiorrhizae	18 g
Radix Achyranthis Bidentatae	12 g
Faeces Vespertilionis	9 g
Radix Ilicis Pubescentis	12 g

Administration: Decoct the above drugs in water for oral dose. One dose daily.

(3) Type of insufficiency of spleen—*Qi*.

Symptoms and Signs: The symptoms and signs of the eye are the same as those of the last type. Other manifestations are pale complexion, listlessness, poor appetite and lassitude, pale tongue with thin fur and weak pulse.

Therapeutic Methods: Invigorating the spleen and replenishing *Qi*.

Recipe: *Buzhong Yiqi Tang* (16)

Ingredients:

Radix Astragali seu Hedysari	15 g
Radix Glycyrrhizae	5 g
Radix Ginseng	10 g
Radix Angelicae Sinensis	10 g
Pericarpium Citri Reticulata	6 g
Rhizoma Cimicifugae	3 g
Radix Bupleuri	3 g
Rhizoma Atractylodis Macrocephalae	10 g

Administration: Decoct the above drugs in water for oral dose. One dose daily.

2. Other therapies

Acupuncture therapy: The commonly used points are Jingming, Qiuhou. Chengqi, Tongziliao, Zangzhu, Ganshu, Shenshu, Pishu, Zusanli, Sanyinjiao etc. Select 3-4 points each time. Once daily or every other day. 10 days is a course.

Ear needling: The selected points are eye 1, eye 2, liver, heart, kidney and gallbladder. Take 3 points each time and retain the needles for more than 30 minutes. Or, apply auricular-plaster therapy.

13.5 Optic Neuritis

Optic neuritis can be classified into papillitis and retrobullar neuritis according to difference of the diseased positions. The disease is usually seen in young and middle aged people. It usually attacks both eyes.

Etiology and Pathogenesis

The disease may be due to: (1) emotional depression and stagnation of liver-Qi, which leads to obstruction of the collaterals; (2) excessive fire of the liver and gallbladder which goes upwards to disturb the lucid orifices; (3) deficiency of liver–*Yin* and kidney–*Yin* which leads to flaring–up of fire of deficiency type; (4) postpartum lactation which leads to deficiency of both *Qi* and blood.

Clinical Manifestations

Papillitis has an acute onset and quick hypopsia until blindness. The fundus examination shows papillary hyperemia and edema with ill–defined margins, obliterated and slight projected physiologic excavation, edema and turbidity of the adjacent retina with small amounts of flame–shaped hemorrhage and greyish white soft exudate spots. The central veins of the retina are filled and tortuous.

Acute retrobulbar neuritis occurs with sudden drop of vision (or even loss of light perception), postbulbar tenderness, sluggish pupillary light reaction. Fundus examination shows no changes of the tissue at the early stage or just slight hyperemia of the optic papilla with blurred margins when pathologic change gets sclose to the optic papilla. The veins are filled. At the late stage, the optic papilla presents a light color or pallor with dumbbell–like scotoma.

Chronic retrobulbar neuritis has a slow drop of vision. There is no change in optic fundus at the early stage. At the late stage, optic atrophy may occur. There is central or paracentral scotoma.

Type and Treatment

1. Internal Treatment

(1) Type of stagnation of liver–*Qi*.

Symptoms and Signs: One of the eye symptoms of Optic Neuritis accompanied by emotional depression which causes dizziness, hypochondriac pain, dry throat, bitter taste and oppressed sensation in the chest.

Therapeutic Method: Relieving the depressed liver.

Recipe: *Xiaoyao San* (83)

Ingredients:

Radix Bupleuri	15 g
Radix Angelicae Sinensis	15 g
Radix Paeoniae Alba	15 g
Rhizoma Atractylodis Macrocephalae	15 g
Poria	15 g
Radix Glycyrrhizae	15 g
Rhizoma Zingiberis Recens	2 slices
Herba Menthae	3 g

Administration: Decoct the above drugs in water for oral dose. One dose daily.

(2) Type of Excessive Fire in the Liver and Gallbladder.

Symptoms and Signs: The affection may involve one eye or both eyes. There is a quick drop of vision or even blindness, accompanied with dizziness, headache, hypochondriac pain and bitter taste in the mouth, flushed face, conjunctival congestion, yellow urine, red margin of tongue and reddened tip, yellow and greasy fur, and wiry, rapid pulse.

Therapeutic Methods: Purging the liver of pathogenic fire.

Recipe: Modified *Longdan Xiegan Tang* (40)

Ingredients:

Radix Gentianae	6 g
Radix Scutellariae	9 g
Fructus Gardeniae	9 g
Rhizoma Alismatis	12 g
Caulis Akebiae	9 g
Semen Plantaginis	9 g

Radix Angelicae Sinensis	3 g
Radix Rehmanniae	9 g
Radix Bupleuri	6 g
Radix Glycyrrhizae	6 g

Administration: Decoct the above drugs in water for oral dose. One dose daily.

(3) Type of hyperactivity of fire due to *Yin* deficiency.

Symptoms and Signs: The symptoms and signs are the same as those of the last type, accompanied with dizziness, tinnitus, deafness, red lips, flushed cheeks, reddened tongue, and wiry, thready and rapid pulse.

Therapeutic Method: Nourishing *Yin* and reducing pathogenic fire.

Recipe: Modified *Zhibai Dihuang Tang* (43)
Ingredients:

Rhizoma Rehmanniae Praeparatae	12 g
Frutus Corni	12 g
Rhizoma Dioscoreae	12 g
Rhizoma Alismatis	9 g
Poria	9 g
Cortex Moutan Radicis	9 g
Rhizoma Anemarrhenae	30 g
Cortex Phellodendri	30 g

Administration: Decoct the above drugs in water for oral dose, one dose daily.

(4) Type of deficiency of both *Qi* and blood.

Symptoms and Signs: The inflammation has been remitted at the late stage of the disease. The optic papilla is a little bit light in color. There is sallow complexion, meagre, mental weariness, pale tongue with thin fur and weak pulse.

Therapeutic Method: Regulating and enriching *Qi* and blood.

Recipe: *Bazhen Tang* (68)
Ingredients:

Radix Angelicae Sinensis	10 g
Rhizoma Ligustici Chuanxiong	5 g
Radix Paeoniae Alba	8 g
Rhizoma Rehmanniae Praeparatae	15 g
Radix Ginseng	3 g
Rhizoma Atractylodis Macrocephalaw Praeparata	10 g
Poria	8 g
Radix Glycyrrhizae	5 g
Rhizoma Zingiberis Recens	3 slices
Fructus Ziziphi Jujubae	2 pieces

Administration: Decoct the above drugs in water for oral dose, one dose daily.

2. Other Therapies

(1) Proprietaries: *Xiaoyao Wan* (111), *Longdan Xiegan Wan* (112), *Zhibai Dihuang Wan* (113) and *Shiquan Dabe Wan* (105) can be respectively used for the cases with the above-mentioned types of the disease after the condition has improved.

(2) Acupuncture therapy: It can be employed along with other therapies. The most frequently used acupoints are Jingming, Qiuhou, Zangzhu, Yuyao, Sizhukong, Fengchi, Sanyinjiao, Neiguang.

(3) Application of hormones during the acute stage may quickly control the development of the disease.

14 Diseases of Vitreous

The vitreous is a colorless, transparent jelly-like substance, filling the vitreous chamber. It is susceptible to the effects of the pathological process of retina and choroid to become opacque. Eye injuries and vitreous retrograde degeneration may also cause opacity, synchysis, posterior detachment, etc, thus resulting in diminution of vision or even blindness. In TCM, the vitreous is termed *Shengao,* falling into the category of pupil. So when vitreous diseases occur, the liver and kidney should be responsible.

14.1 Vitreous Opacity

Vitreous opacity may be caused by internal inflammation, hemorrhage and retragrade products. The main manifestations are muscaegenetic and blurred vision. In TCM, it is termed *Yun Wu Yi Jing.*

Etiology and Pathogenesis

The disease may be due to (1) accumulation and steaming of dampness-heat and attack of turbid *Qi;* (2) stagnation of liver *Qi,* resulting in blood stasis and extravasation; (3) deficiency of the liver and kidney, resulting in flaring up of fire of deficiency type.

Clinical manifestations

In mild cases, black shadows float up and down like flying flies but there is usually no change in vision. In severe cases, the eyes seem to be covered by a membrane, resulting in hyposia or even ablepsia. The examination shows that the appearance of the eyes is normal. Opacity of the vitreous may occur in the form of dust—like, flocky or globular haziness, presenting greyish, yellow or red color. In the examination eye fundus can be clear or blurred or completely invisible, depending upon the degrees of opacity.

Type and Treatment

In the treatment, the cause of the vitreous opacity must be first determined. In accordance with the etiology, we can lay out the treatment.

1. Internal Treatment

(1) Type of accumulation and steaming of dampness—heat.

Symptoms and Signs: Muscaegenetic and blurred vision, vitreous opacity, accompanied with heavy sensation in the head, oppressed sensation in the chest, bitter taste, yellow and greasy fur, and soft, rapid pulse.

Therapeutic Method: Clearing away heat and promoting diuresis.

Recipe: Modified *Sanren Tang* (8)

Ingredients:

Semen Armeniacae Amarum	9 g
Semen Coicis	9 g
Semen Amomi Cardamomi	9 g
Medulla Tetrapanacis	9 g
Herba Lophatheri	9 g
Cortex Magnoliae Officinalis	9 g
Rhizoma Pinelliae	9 g
Talcum	9 g

Radix Paeoniae Rubra	15 g

Modification: For cases with excessive dampness, add:

Semen Plantaginis	9 g
Rhizoma Alismatis	9 g

For cases with excessive heat, add:

Radix Scutellariae	9 g
Fructus Gardeniae	9 g
Flos Lonicerae	24 g

Administration: Decocte the above drugs in water for oral dose, once a day.

(2) Type of stagnation of *Qi* and blood stasis.

Symptoms and Signs: Blurred vision or blindness, hemorrhage in the vitreous presting dust–like or ball–like form, accompanied with emotional depression, oppressed sensation in the chest, fullness in the hypochondria, bitter taste dark red tongue dotted with ecchymosis, white or yellowish fur, and taut and tense or uneven pulse.

Therapeutic Methods: Dispersing the stagnant liver–*Qi*, stopping bleeding and removing blood stasis.

Recipe: Modified *Danzhi Xiaoyao San* (57)

Ingredients:

Cortex Moutan Radicis	9 g
Fructus Gardeniae	9 g
Radix Bupleuri	9 g
Rhizoma Atractylodis Macrocephalae	9 g
Radix Angelicae Sinensis	12 g
Radix Paeoniae Rubra	12 g
Poria	12 g

Modification: For cases with fresh hemorrhage, add:

Herba Agrimoniae	12 g
Herba Ecliptae	12 g
Fresh Pollen Typhae	12 g
Radix Notoginseng	3 g

(to be taken after being infused with the decoction)

For cases with remote hemorrhage, add:

Semen Persicae	9 g
Flos Carthami	9 g
Rhizoma Ligustici Chuanxiong	9 g
Fructus Aurantii	9 g
Radix Curcumae	12 g
Fructus Leonuri	12 g

Administration: Decocte the above drugs in water for oral dose, once a day.

(3) Type of hyperactivity of fire due to *Yin* deficiency.

Symptoms and Signs: Blurred and muscaegenetic vision, dizziness and tinnitus, soreness in the loins and legs, dry mouth and throat, reddened tongue with little fur, and small, rapid pulse.

Therapeutic Method: Nourishing *Yin* and reducing pathogenic fire.

Recipe: Modified *Zhibai Dihuang Tang* (43)

Ingredients:

Rhizoma Anemarrhenae Praeparata	9 g
Cortex Phellodendri Praeparata	9 g
Radix Rehmanniae	9 g
Cortex Moutan Radicis	9 g
Rhizoma Alismatis	9 g
Poria	9 g
Radix Achyranthis Bidentatae	12 g

Radix Paeoniae Rubra	15 g
Radix Ophiopogonis	15 g
Radix Salviae Miltiorrhizae	18 g
Radix Glycyrrhizae	6 g

Administration: Decocte the above drugs in water for oral dose, once a day.

2. Other Therapies

Administration of injection of Radix Salviae Miltiorrhizae (or of Radix Notoginseng or Flos Carthami) through iontophoresis.

15. Orbital Diseases

The causes of the orbital diseases are considerably numerous. TCM therapies can give satisfactory curative effects in treating some intraorbital inflammatory diseases. This chapter will briefly discuss some of them.

15.1 Acute Orbital Inflammation

Generally the onset is sudden with distending pain and exophthalmus. It is usually seen in periorbititis, orbital cellulitis, tenonitis, etc. In TCM, it falls into the category of *Tuqi Jinggao Zheng*.

Etiology and Pathogenesis

It is usually due to the attack of internal heat and pathogenic fire or, due to combined attack of heat and phlegm which accumulates in *Zang-Fu*. Extreme heat, resulting from retention of pathogenic wind in the viscera may also attack the five orbiculi and cause the disease.

Clinical Manifestations

Sudden onset, exophthalmus to varying degrees, red swelling of the eyelid skin, conjunctival congestion, edema, accompanied with limited movement of the globe or completely fixed eyeball, severe ophthalmalgia, and, in severe cases headache, general high fever, nausea, vomiting and potential dangers of secondary panophthalmities, meningitis and cavernous sinus thrombophlebitis.

Type and Treatment

1. Internal Treatment

(1) Type of retention of pathogenic heat.

Symptoms and Signs: The eye symptoms are those mentioned above. Usually, at the beginning of the disease, it is accompanied with fever, aversion to cold, reddened tongue with yellow fur, and rapid or floating, rapid pulse.

Therapeutic Methods: Clearing away fire and toxic materials, promoting blood circulation and eliminating swelling.

Recipe: Combined Prescription of Modified *Xianfang Huoming Yin* (71) and *Wuwei Xiaodu San* (5)

Ingredients In the first recipe:

Squama Manitis	3 g
Radix Trichosanthis	3 g
Radix Glycyrrhizae	3 g
Resina Boswelliae Carterii	3 g
Radix Angelicae Dahuricae	3 g
Radix Paeoniae Rubra	3 g
Bulbus Fritillariae Thunbergii	3 g
Radix Ledebouriellae	3 g
Resina Commiphorae Myrrhae	3 g
Spina Gleditsiae	3 g
The tip of Radix Angelicae Sinensis	3 g
Pericarpium Citri Reticulatae	9 g
Flos Lonicerae	9 g

In the second recipe:

Flos Chrysanthemi Indici	6 g
Herba Taraxaci	6 g
Herba Violae	6 g
Corm seu Herba Begoniae Fimbristipulae	6 g

Administration: Decocte the above drugs in water for oral dose, once a day.

(2) Type of pathogenic heat inside the body.

Symptoms and Signs: The same eye symptoms as those of the last type (but severer), drastic ophthalmagia and headache, accompanied by high fever, polydipsia, flushed face, harsh breath, yellow urine, constipation, scarlet tongue, and rapid, forceful pulse, etc.

Therapeutic Method: Clearing away heat and toxic materials in *Ying* system.

Recipe: Modified *Qingying Tang* (4)

Ingredients:

Cornu Rhinoceri	2 g
Radix Rehmanniae	15 g
Radix Scrophulariae	9 g
Leaves bud of Herba Lophatheri	3 g
Radix Ophiopogonis	9 g
Radix Salviae Miltiorrhizae	6 g
Rhizoma Coptidis	5 g
Flos Lonicerae	9 g
Fructus Forsythiae	6 g

Administration: Decoct the above drugs in water for oral dose, once a day.

2. Other Therapies

(1) Type of external treatment: Smash Allium Fistulosum and mugwort leaf and get them heated and packed in a piece of cloth and apply them to the affected part for hot compress.

(2) Radix Angelicae Dahuricae, Herba Asari, Radix Angelicae Sinensis, Rhizoma Atractylodis, Herba Ephedrae,

Radix Ledebouriellae, Rhizoma seu Radix Notopterygii

Decoct the drugs in water. Use the decoction to fumigate and wash the eye locally.

(3) Those who have pus may be given local incision to discharge pus.

(4) Antibiotics may be used for acute and severe cases.

15.2　Orbital Pseudotumor

This disease is a nonspecific chronic proliferative inflammation with unknown etiology. It can induce exophthalmus and ocular dysinesia, and usually affects one eye. Males are affected more often than females. The differentiation between pseudotumor and tumor should be made. In TCM, it is termed *Guyan Ningjing Zheng*.

Etiology and Pathogenesis

The disease is due to wind and heat as pathogen which attack the head and eyes leading to stagnation and obstruction of ocular vessels, stagnancy of *Qi* and blood; long standing hyperactivity of pathogenic heat will impair and consume *Yin* fluid and cause sluggishness of blood circulation and stagnation of *Qi* and blood, thus resulting in the disease.

Clinical Manifestations

There is exophthalmus, ocular dyscinesia, and in above half of the cases inflammation, ophthalmalgia, conjunctival congestion and hydrops. In most of the patients, a fixed mass with indistinct boundary can be palpated with tenderness. In severe cases the orbit may be filled by the mass. At the early stage, usually no changes occur in visual acuity and ocular fundus. At the late stage, in very few cases, retro-ocular polar may be oppressed.

Type and Treatment

1. Internal Treatment

(1) Type of excessiveness of pathogenic wind-heat and obstruction of the ocular vessels.

Symptoms and Signs: Exophthalmus, bulbar conjunctival congestion, limited eye movement, accompanied with general symptoms such as headache, stiffness of neck, flushed face, fever, etc. The patient has a reddened tongue with yellowish coating and rapid pulse.

Therapeutic Method: Dispelling pathogenic wind, clearing away heat and toxic materials, promoting blood circulation and removing obstruction in the vessels.

Recipe: Modified *Xienao Tang* (72)

Ingredients:

Radix Scutellariae	9 g
Radix et Rhizoma Rhei	6 g
Natrii Sulfas Exsiccatus	3 g
Semen Plantaginis	9 g
Caulis Akebiae	6 g
Poria	9 g
Radix Ledebouriellae	6 g
Radix Platycodi	9 g
Fructus Leonuri	12 g
Radix Scrophulariae	12 g
Rhizoma Coptidis	6 g
Radix Paeoniae Rubra	12 g
Radix Angelicae Sinensis	12 g

Administration: Decoct the above drugs in water for oral dose once a day.

(2) Type of prolonged excessiveness of pathogenic heat causing blood stasis and *Yin*-deficiency.

Symptoms and Signs: The same ocular symptoms as those of the above type, accompanied by dizziness, tinnitus, dysphoria with feverish sensation in the palms and sores, palpitation and insomnia, thin physique, dark red tongue, wiry, small and uneven pulse, etc.

Therapeutic Method: Nourishing *Yin* and clearing away heat, removing blood stasis and resolving the mass.

Recipe: Modified *Tongyou Tang* (73)

Ingredients:

Rhizoma Rehmanniae Preaparatae	9 g
Radix Glycyrrhizae Praeparata	3 g
Radix Angelicae Sinensis	6 g
Flos Carthami	3 g
Semen Persicae	12 g
Radix Rehmanniae	9 g
Fructus Ligustri Lucidi	12 g
Herba Ecliptae	15 g
Plastrum Testudinis	12 g
Carapax Trionycis	12 g
Spica Prunellae	15 g
Concha Ostreae	15 g

Administration: Decoct the above drugs in water for oral dose, once a day.

2. Other Therapies

(1) Apart from TCM therapies, antibiotics and hormones may be used.

(2) Radiotherapy is suitable to those with lymphocytotic

predominance.

(3) Prick Yingxiang, Taiyang, Shangxing and upper eyelid with a three-edged needle and squeeze out blood so as to remove stagnancy and reduce excessiveness of pathogenic heat.

16 Disorders of Ocular Muscles

Strabismus refers to the deviation of the eye, including concomitant and non-concomitant strabismus. It is the main pathogenic factor for binocular visual disturbance. Amblyopia will be caused as a result of protracted restriction of movement of the deviating eye.

16.1 Paralytic Strabismus

Paralytic strabismus can be divided into congenital strabismus and acquired strabismus. Due to congenital dysplasis, congenital strabismus is mainly treated with surgical operation. This chapter will only discuss the acquired strabismus. Because of the injuries to the nerves and muscles, acquired strabismus is characterized by limited eye movement, deviation of the eye and diplopia. In TCM, it is known as *Feng Qian Pian Shi*.

Etiology and Pathogenesis

Paralytic strabismus usually results from deficiency of vital *Qi*, weakness of *wei-Qi*, and direct invasion into the channels and collaterals by pathogenic wind and heat. If a person has accumulated dampness and phlegm caused by dysfunction of the spleen in transportation of aqueous liquids, he / she will be vulnerable to the disease when attacked by exogenous pathogenic wind because the phlegm and wind tend to collabuate to obstruct the passage of the channels in the ocular muscles. Besides, malnutrition of the muscles and tendons of the eye due to deficiency of *Qi* and blood may also lead to the disease.

Clinical Manifestations

Paralytic strabismus usually has a sudden onset, deviation of the eye, and limited movement of the eyeball. In most cases, it attacks one of the eyes. The patient experiences diplopia caused by sudden damage of binocular vision, dizziness, nausea or vomiting. After a period of time, the paralyzed eyes may return to normal, or result in monocular inhibition, and diplopia may disappear.

Type and Treatment

1. Internal Treatment

(1) Type of invasion into the collaterals by pathogenic wind.

Symptoms and Signs: Sudden deviation of the eyeball, limited eye movement, diplopia, headache, aversion to cold, fever, thin and whitish fur, and floating pulse.

Therapeutic Methods: Dispersing pathogenic wind and dredging the channel

Recipe: Modified *Xiao Xu Ming Tang* (74)

Ingredients:

Herba Ephedrae	9 g
Radix Ledebouriellae	9 g
Radix Stephaniae Tetrandrae	9 g
Radix Aconiti Praeparata	9 g
Rhizoma Zingiberis Recens	9 g
Rhizoma Ligustici Chuanxiong	9 g
Radix Paeoniae Alba	15 g
Radix Codonopsis Pilosulae	15 g
Radix Puerariae	15 g
Radix Scutellariae	6 g

| Radix Glycyrrhizae | 6 g |

Administration: Decoct the above drugs in water for oral dose. Once a day.

(2) Type of obstruction of collaterals by wind and phlegm.

Symptoms and Signs: Besides the eye symptoms of the last type mentioned above, there is anorexia, profuse phlegm, thick and greasy fur, and wiry and smooth pulse.

Therapeutic Methods: Strengthening the spleen and reducing phlegm, despelling wind and removing obstruction in the channel

Recipe: *Liu JunZi Tang* (75) and *Zheng Rong Tang* (76)

Ingredients:

Poria	9 g
Rhizoma Atractylodis Marcocephalae	9 g
Rhizoma Pinelliae	9 g
Rhizoma Typhonii	9 g
Bombyx Batryticatus	9 g
Rhizoma seu Radix Notopterygii	9 g
Radix Ledebouriellae	9 g
Radix Paeoniae Rubra	15 g
Radix Codonopsis Pilosulae	15 g
Ramulus Uncariae cum Uncis	15 g
Radix Glycyrrhizae	6 g

Administration: Decoct the above drugs in water for oral dose. One dose daily.

(3) Type of deficieny of *Qi* and blood.

Symptoms and Signs: All the eye symptoms are the same as those of the types mentioned above. There is also hemiplegia, sallow complexion, pale tongue, whitish fur and weak pulse.

Therapeutic Method: Nourishing *Qi* and blood

Recipe: Modified *Buyang Huanwu Tang* (77)

Ingredients:

Semen Persicae	9 g
Flos Carthami	9 g
Rhizoma Ligustici Chuanxiong	9 g
tip of Radix Angellicae Sinensis	9 g
Rhizoma Typhonii	9 g
Bombyx Batryticatus	9 g
Radix Puerariae	9 g
Radix Astragali seu Hedysari	15 g
Radix Paeoniae Rubra	15 g
Concha Haliotidis	15 g
Lumbricus	15 g

Administration: Decoct the above drugs in water for oral dose. Once a day.

2. Other Therapies

(1) Acupuncture: Usually the selected points are: Tongziliao, Chengqi, Jiache, Dicang, Taiyang, Qianzheng, Hegu, Taichong, etc. Needle 3 local points and 2 distal points a time, once a day.

(2) Moxibustion: Apply moxibustion to some of the points mentioned above.

(3) Intramuscular injection with vitamin B_1 and vitamin B_{12}.

16.2 Concomitant Strabismus

Concomitant strabismus is a manifest deviation from parallelism of the two eyes; the angle of deviation is the same in all fields of gaze. In TCM, concomitant strabismus is termed *Xiao Er Tong Jing*.

Etiology and Pathogenesis

Tendons and meridians of children are tender. When they are invaded by exogenous pathogenic wind and heat, the channels are often injured, causing stagnation of *Qi*. Hence the disease. Besides, the disease can also result from stagnation of *Qi* and blood stasis caused by fright or trauma which, too, impairs the channels.

Clinical Manifestations

The concomitant strabismus occurs characteristically at the age of three. The deviation of the eyeball may be horizontal or vertical, and clinically, horizontal deviation is more often seen. There is no limitation of eye movement. The eyeball can move freely in all directions while the angle of deviation is always the same. Due to long-standing inhibition, the deviating eye may result in amblyopia but not diplopia. However, alternating strabismus will not develop into amblyopia.

Type and Treatment

At the early stage, treatment will have better results. If amblyopia is formed, the treatment should be based on nourishing the liver and kidney, and reprenishing *Qi* and blood.

1. Internal Treatment

(1) If the meridians are obstructed by flaming-up of pathogenic wind-heat, dispersing wind-heat, dredging meridians by activating blood circulation should be considered.

Recipe: *Longdan Xuegan Tang* (40) and *Taohong Siwu Tang* (78)

Ingredients:

Radix Gentianae	9 g
Radix Scutellariae	9 g
Fructus Gardeniae	9 g

Radix Bupleuri	9 g
Semen Plantaginis	9 g
Radix Rehmanniae	15 g
Radix Angelicae Sinensis	15 g
Radix Paeoniae Rubra	15 g
Semen Persicae Praeparata	6 g
Flos Carthami	6 g

Administration: Decoct the above drugs in water for oral dose, once a day.

(2) For stagnation of *Qi* and blood resulting from sudden fright, tranquilizing the mind, relieving muscular spasm, and activating and nourishing blood should be considered.

Recipe: Modified *Anshen Zhinjing Wan* (116)

Ingredients:

Radix Codonopsis Pilosulae	9 g
Lignum Pini Poriaferum	9 g
Radix Ophiopogonis	9 g
Radix Angelicae Sinensis	9 g
Herba Menthae	9 g
Rhizoma Coptidis	9 g
Fructus Gardeniae	9 g
Radix Rehmanniae	15 g
Radix Paeoniae Rubra	15 g
Semen Ziziphi Spinosae Praeparata	30 g
Semen Biotae	18 g

Administration: Decoct the above drugs in water for oral dose, one dose daily.

(3) For injuries to the tendons and meridians by trauma, activating blood circulation to remove blood stasis, and eliminating

phlegm to dredge the meridians should be considered.

Recipe: Modified *Tong Xue Wan* (79)

Ingredients:

Herba Schizonepetae	9 g
Radix Ledebouriellae	9 g
Rhizoma seu Radix Notopterygi	9 g
Rhizoma Ligustici	9 g
Rhizoma Ligustici Chuanxiong	9 g
Pericarpium Citri Reticulatae	9 g
Rhizoma Pinelliae	9 g
Arisaema cum Bile	9 g
Radix Paeoniae Rugra	15 g
Radix Angelicae Sinensis	15 g
Radix Rehmanniae	15 g

Administration: Decoct the above drugs in water for oral dose, one dose daily.

2. Other Therapies

(1) If medicines fail to produce good effect as expected, operation should be performed as early as possible.

(2) If amblyopia has developed to a severe degree, pleoptecs can be used as an auxiliary therapeutic method.

17 Ocular Trauma

Ocular trauma refers to injuries of the eyeball and its surrounding tissues caused by exogenous factors. This chapter will mainly discuss the contusion and penetrating injuries to the eyes.

17.1 Contusion Injuries

Contusion injuries are commonly produced by a direct blow to the eye with a blunt object which causes a series of injuries. It belongs to the category of contusion wounds in the ophthalmology of TCM.

Etiology and Pathogenesis

A direct blow to the eye with a blunt object (such as a ball, a piece of wood or stone, a brick or tile, a belt, a stick and a piece of iron) may injure the eyelid and the tissues in the eyeball.

Clinical Manifestations

The possible results of contusion injuries are edema of the lids, ecchymoma, conjunctival edema, congestion, corneal abrasions and exuviation. A severe injury may cause eyeball rupture, hyphema, iridodiastasis, mydriasis, dislocation of the crystalline lens, hemorrhage into the vitreous, rupture of the choroid, retinal hemorrhage and detachment, exudation and edema at the macula retinae.

Type and Treatment

1. Internal Treatment

(1) Hemorrhage of the traumatic choroid.

Symptoms and Signs: Cyanosis and swelling of the eyelids, heavy sensation of the eye, inability to open the eyelids, or intraobital blood stasis and exophthalmus; or subconjunctival ecchymosis, or hyphema, or hemorrhage in the fundus.

Therapeutic Methods: Stopping bleeding and activating the blood

Recipe: Modified *Shihui San* (80)
 Herba seu Radix Cirsii Japonici
 Herba Cephalanoploris
 Folium Nelumbinis
 Cacumen Biotae
 Rhizoma Imperatae
 Radix Rubiae
 Fructus Gardeniae
 Radix et Rhizoma Rhei
 Cortex Moutan Radicis
 Petiolus Trachycarpi

Char equal shares of the drugs without altering their property and grind them into fine powder. Pound Lotus roots into juice and mix it with the powder. Take the mixture after meals, 15 g a time.

After hemostasis, activating blood circulation to dissipate blood stasis should be considered.

Recipe: *Qu Yu Tang* (70)

Lateral Root Angelicae Sinensis	12 g
Radix Paeoniae Eubra	12 g
Semen Persicae	9 g
Herba Lycopi	9 g
Radix Salviae Miltiorrhizae	15 g

Rhizoma Ligustici Chuanxiong	6 g
Radix Curcumae	12 g
Radix Rehmanniae	12 g
Herba Ecliptae	12 g
Herba Agrimoniae	12 g

Decoct the drugs in water for oral dose. Take one dose daily.

(2) *Qi*-stagnation and blood stasis.

Symptoms and Signs: There is a complaint of discomfort in the eye with blurred vision. The examination shows turbidity of the lens and vitreous, retinal edema, and stabbing and distending pain in the eye.

Therapeutic Method: Activating *Qi* and blood circulation, removing blood stasis and relieving pain.

Recipe: Modified *Taohong Siwu Tang* (78)

Rhizoma Rehmanniae Praeparatae	12 g
Rhizoma Ligustici Chuanxiong	9 g
Radix Paeoniae Alba	12 g
Radix Angelicae Sinensis	12 g
Semen Persicae	6 g
Flos Carthami	6 g
Cortex Moutan Radicis	12 g
Radix Salviae Miltiorrhizae	15 g
Radix Curcumiae	12 g
Fructus Aurantii	6 g

Decoct the drugs in water for oral dose, one dose daily.

2. Other Therapies

(1) Propietary: *Qiju Dihuang Wan* (110) for oral administration

It is used at the late stage to improve vision. Take two

boluses, 18 g each time, twice a day.

(2) If an injury is so severe as to cause serious blood stasis in the anterior chamber and vitreous, the patient should lie in bed with both eyes covered with eye pad and accept the therapy of ion—introduction with the solution of Radix Notoginseng or Radix Salviae Mitiorrhizae.

(3) In cases with laceration or escape of the contents of the eyeball, the wound should be repaired. Measures must be taken to prevent infections.

17.2　Penetrating Injuries to the Eye

Penetrating injuries are usually caused by small, sharp object perforating the globe, or bits of metals, crushed stone, or shell fragments flying into the eye. The patient's condition depends on the location of the wounds, cause and degree. It also depends on whether there is foreign body remaining within the eyeball and the prsence or absence of infection. This disease belongs to the category of *Zhenjing Posun* in the ophthalmology of TCM.

Etiology and Pathogonesis

The eyeball has been penetrated by a knife, scissors, an awl, a needle or by high-speed flying particles of metal, crushed stone, shell fragments.

Clinical Manifestations

The injuried eyes may differ in degree in pain, photophobia, lacrimation, lid spasm and visual disturbance. The injury may cause perforation of cornea, laceration of bulbar conunctiva, escape of aqueous humor. The anterior chamber becomes shallow or vanished. There is also hyphema, irregularity of the pupil and luxation of the lens, or rupture of the lens capsule. An severe injury may cause escape of the contents of the eyeball, deformation of the eyeball, leading to blindness.

For penetrating injuries, it is necessary to observe whether or not there is secondary infections, foreign body remaining in the eye, and the occurence of sympathetic ophthalmia.

Type and Treatment

1. Internal Treatment

(1) Type of *Qi* stagnation and blood stasis.

Symptoms and Signs: Laceration of the ocular tissues, serious pains of the eyeball, hyperemia, photophobia and lacrimation.

Therapeutic Method: Activating blood circulation, dissipating blood stasis and dispelling wind.

Recipe: *Chufeng Yisun Tang* (55)

Radix Angelicae Sinensis	6 g
Radix Paeoniae Alba	6 g
Rhizoma Rehmanniae Praeparatae	6 g
Rhizoma Ligustici Chuangxiong	6 g
Rhizoma Ligustici	5 g
Radix Peucedani	5 g
Radix Ledebouriellae	5 g

Modifications: For cases with opacity of the cornea,

add: Herba Equiseti Hiemalis	6 g
Periostracum Cicadae	9 g
Flos Chrysanthemi	9 g

For cases with edema of the ocular fundus,

add: Rhizoma Alismatis	12 g
Semen Plantaginis	9 g
Poria	9 g

For cases with photophobia and lacrimation,
add: Rhizoma seu Radix Notopterygii 6 g
Herba Menthae 6 g
Radix Gentianae 9 g
For cases with serious pain of the eye,
add: Resina Boswelliae Carterii 6 g
Resina Commiphorae Myrrhae 6 g

Decoct the herbs in water. Take one dose daily, three times a day.

(2) Type of hemorrhage of the traumatic choroid.

Symptoms and Signs: Subconjunctiva ecchymosis or hyphema or ocular fundus hemorrhage.

Therapeutic Method: Cooling the blood and stopping bleeding.

Recipe: *Shihui San* (80)

Ingredients: Herba seu Radix Cirsii Japonici
Herba Cephalanoploris
Colium Nelumbinis
Cacumen Biotae
Rhizoma Imperatae
Radix Rubiae
Fructus Gardeniae
Radix et Rhizoma Rhei
Cortex Moutan Radicis
Patiolus Trachycarpi

Char equal shares of the drugs without altering their property and grind them into fine powder. Pound Lotus roots into juice and mix it with the powder. Take the mixture after meals, 15 g a time, three times a day.

(3) Type of excessiveness of pathagenic evils.

Symptoms and Signs: Sharp pain in the eye, swelling of the wound, hypopyon or even panophthalmia.

Therapeutic Method: Clearing away heat and toxic materials, cooling and activating the blood.

Recipe: *Wuwei Qingdu Yin* (5) and *Xijiao Dihuang Tan* (81)

Flos Lonicerae	9 g
Flos Chrysanthemi Indici	6 g
Herba Taraxaci	6 g
Herba Violae	6 g
Herba Senecio Nudicaulis	6 g
Cornu Rhinoceri	3 g
Radix Rehmanniae	30 g
Radix Paeoniae	12 g
Cortex Moutan Radicis	9 g

Decoct the herbs in water for oral does. Take one dose daily, three times a day.

2. Other Therapies

(1) Perform debridement and saturing as early as possible, remove any foreign bodies and prevent infection.

(2) If necessary, inject tetanus antitoxin to prevent tetanus.

(3) Locally use 0.5% Atropine as mydriatic, and 0.5% Cortisone and antibiotic eye drops for instillation.

Appendix

1. *Yinqiao San*
Source: *Wenbing Tiabian* (Treatise on Differentiation and Treatment of Epidemic Febrile Diseases).
Flos Lonicerae
Fructus Forsythiae
Radix Platycodi
Herba Menthae
Herba Lophatheri
Spica Schizonepetae
Radix Glycyrrhizae
Semen Sojae Praetaratum
Fructus Arctii
Rhizoma Phragmitis

2. *Neishu Huanglian Tang*
Source: *Yizong Jinjian* (The Golden Mirror of Medicine)
Fructus Gardeniae
Fructus Forsythiae
Herba Menthae
Radix Glycyrrhizae
Radix Scutellariae
Rhizoma Coptidis
Radix Platycodi
Radix et Rhizoma Rhei

Radix Angelicae Sinensis
Radix Paeoniae Alba
Radix Aucklandiae
Semen Arecae

3. *Puji Xiaodu Yin*
Source: *Mujing Dacheng* (A book written by Huang Ting-jing in 1748)
Radix Scutellariae
Rhizoma Coptidis
Pericarpium Citri Reticulatae
Radix Glycyrrhizae
Radix Scrophulariae
Fructus Forsythiae
Radix Isatidis
Lasiosphaera seu Calvatia
Fructus Arctii
Herba Menthae
Radix Bupleuri
Bombyx Batryticatus
Rhizoma Cimicifugae
Radix Platycodi

4. *Qingying Tang*
Source: *Wenbing Tiaobian* (Treatise on Differentiation and Treatment of Epidemic Febrile Diseases)
Cornu Rhinoceri
Radix Scrophulariae
Radix Ophiopogonis

Flos Lonicerae
Radix Rehmanniae
Radix Salviae Miltiorrhizae
Fructus Forsythiae
Rhizoma Coptidis
Leaves bud of Herba Lophatheri

5. *Wuwei Xiaodu Yin*
Source: *Yizong Jinjian* (The Golden Mirror of Medicine)
Flos Lonicerae
Flos Chrysanthemi Indici
Herba Taraxaci
Herba Violae
Herba Senecio Nudicaulis

6. *Sanre Xiaodu Yinzi*
Source: *Shenshi Yaohan* (A Valuable Manual of Ophthalmology)
Rhizoma Coptidis
Radix Scutellariae
Fructus Forsythiae
Fructus Arctii
Herba Menthae
Rhizoma seu Radix Notopterygii
Radix Ledebouriellae

7. *Huanglian Jiedu Tang*
Source: *Waitai Miyao* (The Medical Secrets of an Official)
Radix Scutellariae

Rhizoma Coptidis
Cortex Phellodendri
Fructus Gardeniae

8. *Sanren Tang*
Source: *Wenbing Tiaobian* (Treatise on Differentiation and Treatment of Epidemic Febrile Diseases)
Semen Armeniacae Amarum
Talcum
Medulla Tetrapanacis
Herba Lophatheri
Cortex Magnoliae Officinalis
Semen Coicis
Rhizoma Pinelliae
Semen Amomi Cardamomi

9. *Chushi Tang*
Source: *Yanke Zuanyao* (A book written by Huang Yan in 1867)
Fructus Forsythiae
Talcum
Semen Plantaginis
Fructus Aurantii
Radix Scutellariae
Rhizoma Coptidis
Caulis Akebiae
Radix Glycyrrhizae
Pericarpium Citri Reticulatae
Herba Schizonepetae

Poria
Radix Ledebouriellae

10. *Siwu Tang* **with modifications**
Source: *Shenshi Yaohan* (A Valuable Manual of Ophthalmology)
Radix Sophorae Flavescentis
Herba Menthae
Rhizoma Ligustici Chuanxiong
Radix Rehmanniae
Fructus Arctii
Fructus Forsythiae
Radix Trichosanthis
Radix Ledebouriellae
Radix Paeoniae Rubra
Radix Angelicae Sinensis
Spica Schizonepetae

11. *Huajian Ercheng Wan*
Source: *Yizong Jinjian* (The Golden Mirror of Medicine)
Pericarpium Citri Reticulatae
Rhizoma Pinelliae Praeparatae
Poria
Radix Glycyrrhizae
Bombyx Batryticatus Alba
Rhizoma Coptidis

12. *Fangfeng Sanjie Tang*
Source: *Mujing Dacheng* (A book written by Huang

Ting-jing in 1748)
Herba Schizonepetae
Radix Ledebouriellae
Radix Angelicae Pubescentis
Flos Carthami
Lignum Sappan
Radix Angelicae Sinensis
Herba Dendrobii
Pollen Typhae
Talcum
Cortex Mori Radicis
Excrementa Bombycum
Rhizoma Smilacis Glabrae
Radix Paeoniae Alba

13. *Zaoshi Tang*
Source: *Shenshi Yaohan* (A Valuable Manual of Ophthalmology)
Rhizoma Coptidis
Rhizoma Atractylodis
Rhizoma Atractylodis Macrocephalae
Pericarpium Citri Reticulatae
Poria
Rhizoma Pinelliae
Fructus Aurantii
Fructus Cardeniae
Radix Glycyrrhizae

14. *Chaihu San*

Source: *Shenshi Yaohan* (A Valuable Manual of Ophthalmology)
Radix Bupleuri
Radix Ledebouriellae
Radix Paeoniae Rubra
Herba Schizonepetae
Rhizoma seu Radix Notopterygii
Radix Platycodi
Radix Rehmanniae
Radix Glycyrrhizae

15. *Huangqi Tang*
Source: *Michuan Yanke Longmu Lum* (Long Mu's Secret Treatise on Ophthalmology)
Radix Astragali seu Hedysari
Fructus Leonuri
Radix Ledebouriellae
Cortex Lycii Radicis
Poria
Radix et Rhizoma Rhei
Radix Ginseng
Radix Scutellariae
Radix Glycyrrhizae

16. *Buzhong Yiqi Tang*
Source: *Dongheng Shishu* (A book written by Wang Xi-jin in early 15th century)
Radix Astragali seu Hedysari
Radix Glycyrrhizae Praeparata

Radix Codonopsis Pilosulae
Radix Angelicae Sinensis
Percarpium Citri Reticulatae
Rhizoma Cimicifugae
Radix Bupleuri
Rhizoma Atractylodis Macrocephalae

17. *Zhuyang Huoxie Tang*
Source: *Zhenghi Zhunsheng* (Standards of Diagnosis and Treatment)
Radix Astragali seu Hedysari
Radix Glycyrrhizae Praeparata
Radix Ledebouriellae
Radix Angelicae Sinensis
Radix Angelicae Dahuricae
Fructus Viticis
Rhizoma Cimicifugae
Radix Bupleuri

18. *Shengqi Wan*
Source: *Jinkui Yaolue* (Synopsis of Prescriptions of the Golden Chamber)
Radix Rehmanniae Praeparata
Rhizoma Dioscoreae
Fructus Corni
Cortex Moutan Radicis
Rhizoma Alismatis
Poria
Radix Aconiti Praeparata

Cortex Cinnamomi

19. *Zhilei Bugan Tang*
Source: *Yiahong Jinjian* (The Golden Mirror of Medicien)
Radix Angelicae Sinensis
Radix Rehmanniae Praeparata
Rhizoma Ligustici Chuanxiong
Radix Paeoniae Alba
Fructus Tribuli Alba
Herba Equiseti Hiemalis
Radix Ledebouriellae

20. *Xiepi Chure Yin*
Source: *Yinhai Jingwei* (Essence of Silvery Sea)
Radix Astragali seu Hedysari
Radix Ledebouriellae
Fructus Leonuri
Radix Platycodi
Radix et Rhizoma Rhei
Rhizoma Coptidis
Radix Scutellariae
Semen Plantaginis
Natrii Sulfas

21. *Qianjin Tuoli San*
Source: *Yanke Jicheng* (A book written by Cheng Shan-tang in 1820)
Radix Codonopsis Pilosulae
Fresh Radix Astragali seu Hedysari

Poria
Radix Glycyrrhizae
Radix Angelicae Sinensis
Radix Paeoniae Alba
Rhizoma Ligustici Chuanxiong
Radix Platycodi
Flos Lonicerae
Radix Angelicae Dahuricae
Radix Ledebouriellae
Radix Ophiopogonis

22. *Zhuye Xiejing Tang*
Source: *Yuanji Qiwei* (Revealing the Mystery of the Origin of Eye Diseases)
Radix Bupleuri
Fructus Gardeniae
Rhizoma seu Radix Notopterygii
Rhizoma Cimicifugae
Radix Glycyrrhizae Praeparata
Radix Scutellariae
Rhizoma Coptidis
Radix et Rhizoma Rhei
Poria
Radix Paeoniae Rubra
Rhizoma Alismatis
Semen Cassiae
Semen Plantaginis
Herba Lophatheri

23. *Chufeng Qingpi Yin*
Source: *Shenshi Yaohan* (A Valuable Manual of Ophthalmology)
Pericarpium Citri Reticulatae
Fructus Forsythiae
Radix Ledebouriellae
Rhizoma Anemarrhenae
Natrii Sulfas Exsiccatus
Radix Scutellariae
Radix Scrophulariae
Rhizoma Coptidis
Spica Schizonepetae
Radix et Rhizoma Rhei
Radix Platycodi
Radix Rehmanniae

24. *Qingpi Liangxue Tang*
Source: *Yizong Jinjian* (The Golden Mirror of Medicine)
Pericarpium Citri Reticulatae
Rhizoma Atractylodis
Cortex Dictamni Radicis
Cortex Magnoliae Officinalis
Radix Paeoniae Rubra
Radix et Rnizoma Rhei
Fructus Forcythiae
Periostracum Cicadae
Herba Schizonepetae
Radix Ledebouriellae
Herba Lophatheri

Radix Glycyrrhizae
Radix Scrophulariae

25. *Guishao Honghua San*
Source: *Shenshi Yaohan* (A Valuable Manual of Ophthalmology)
Radix Angelicae Sinensis
Radix et Rhizoma Rhei
Fructus Gardeniae
Radix Scutellariae
Flos Carthami
Radix Paeoniae Rubra
Radix Glycyrrhizae
Radix Angelicae Dahuricae
Radix Ledebouriellae
Fructus Forsythiae
Radix Rehmanniae

26. *Qufeng Sanre Yinzi*
Source: *Shenshi Yaohan* (A Valuable Manual of Ophthalmology)
Fructus Forsythiae
Fructus Arctii
Rhizoma seu Radix Notopterygii
Herba Menthae
Radix et Rhizoma Rhei
Radix Paeoniae Rubra
Radix Ledebouriellae
The Tip of Radix Angelicae Sinensis

Radix Glycyrrhizae
Fructus Gardeniae
Rhizoma Ligustici Chuanxiong

27. *Xiefei Yin*
Source: *Yanke Zuanyao* (A book written by Huang Yan in 1867)
Gypsum Fibrosum
Radix Paeoniae Rubra
Radix Scutellariae
Crotex Mori Radicis
Fructus Aurantii
Caulis Akebiae
Fructus Forsythiae
Herba Schizonepetae
Radix Ledebouriellae
Fructus Gardeniae
Radix Angelicae Dahuricae
Rhizoma sue Radix Notopterygii
Radix Glycyrrhizae

28. *Qinggan San*
Source: *Shenshi Yaohan* (A Valuable Manual of Ophthalmology)
The Tip of Radix Angelicae Sinensis
Rhizoma Ligustisi Chanxiong
Herba Menthae
Radix Rehmanniae
Rhizoma seu Radix Notopterygii

Fructus Gardeniae
Radix et Rhizoma Rhei
Radix Gentianae
Radix Ledebouriellae
Radix Glycyrrhizae

29. *Qingwen Baidu Yin*
Source: *Yizhen Yide* (A View of Epidemic Febrile Diseases With Rashes)
Gypsum Fibrosum
Radix Rehmanniae
Cornu Saigae Tatariace
Rhizoma Coptidis
Radix Scutellariae
Fructus Gardeniae
Radix Platycodi
Rhizoma Anemarrhenae
Radix Paeoniae Rubra
Fructus Forsythiae
Radix Scrophulariae
Fructus Glycyrrizae
Cortex Moutan Radicis
Herba Lophatheri

30. *Sangbaipi Tang*
Source: *Shenshi Yaohan* (A Valuable Manual of Ophthalmology)
Cortex Mori Radicis
Rhizoma Alismatis

Radix Scrophulariae
Radix Glycyrrhizae
Radix Ophiopogonis
Radix Scutellariae
Flos Inulae
Flos Chrysanthemi
Cortex Lycii Radicis
Radix Platycodi
Poria

31. *Xiefei Tang*
Source: *Shenshi Yaohan* (A Valuable Manual of Ophthalmology)
Cortex Mori Radicis
Radix Scutellariae
Cortex Lycii Radicis
Rhizoma Anemarrhenae
Radix Ophiopogonis
Radix Platycodi

32. *Qingzao Jiufei Tang*
Source: *Yimen Falu* (Principles and Prohibitions for Medical Profession)
Folium Mori
Gypsum Fibrosum
Fructus Cannabis
Radix Ophiopogonis
Colla Corii Asini
Folium Eriobotryae

Semen Armeniacae Amarum
Radix Codonopsis Pilosulae
Radix Glycyrrhizae

33. *Yejin Tang*
Source: *Mujing Dacheng* (A book written by Huang Ting-jing in 1748)
Radix Scrophulariae
Cortex Mori Radicis
Fructus Aurantii
Rhizoma Coptidis
Semen Armeniacae Amarum
Flos Inulae
Radix Ledebouriellae
Radix Scutellariae
Flos Chrysanthemi
Semen Lepidii seu Descurainiae

34. *Xiaofeng Chure Tang*
Source: *Yanke Jicheng* (A book written by Cheng Santang in 1820)
Radix Bupleuri
Radix Peucedani
Herba Schizonepetae
Radix Ledebouriellae
Radix Angelicae Dahuricae
Herba Menthae
Radix Gentianae
Radix et Rhizoma Rhei

Radix Puerariae
Gypsum Fibrosum
Radix Glycyrrhizae
Radix Scutellariae

35. *Dangui Huoxie Yin*
Source: *Shenshi Yaohan* (A Valuable Manual of Ophthalmology)
Radix Angelicae Sinensis
Radix Rehmanniae Praeparata
Radix Paeoniae Alba
Rhizoma Ligustici Chuanxiong
Rhizoma seu Radix Notopterygii
Herba Menthae
Herba Astragali seu Hedysari
Radix Ledebouriellae
Rhizoma Atractylodis
Radix Glycyrrhizae

36. *Xiexing Tang*
Source: *Yanke Zuanyao* (A book written by Huang Yan in 1867)
Rhizoma Coptidis
Radix Rehmanniae
Fructus Forsythiae
Radix Paeoniae Rubra
The Tip of Radix Angelicae Sinensis
Semen Plantaginis
Herba Schizonepetae

Radix Ledebouriellae
Fructus Aurantii
Radix Glycyrrhizae
Gypsum Fibrosum

37. *Ziyin Jianghuo Tang*
Source: *Shenshi Yaohan* (A Valuable Manual of Ophthalmology)
Radix Rehmanniae
Radix Ophiopogonis
Rhizoma Anemarrhenae
Cortex Phellodendri
Radix Scutellariae
Herba Angelicae Sinensis
Rhizoma Ligustici Chuanxiong
Radix Rehmanniae Praeparatae
Radix Paeoniae Alba
Radix Bupleuri
Radix Glycyrrhizae

38. *Sanfeng Chushi Huoxie Tang*
Source: *Zhongyi Yanke Linchuang Shijian* (A book written by Pang Zan-xiang in 1975)
Rhizoma seu Radix Notopterygii
Radix Angelicae Pubescentis
Radix Ledebouriellae
Radix Peucedani
Radix Angelicae Sinensis
Rhizoma Ligustici Chuanxiong

Radix Paeoniae Rubra
Flos Carthami
Caulis Spatholobi
Caulis Lonicerae
Rhizoma Atractylodis
Rhizoma Atractylodis Macrocephalae
Fructus Aurantii
Radix Glycyrrhizae

39. *Xinzhi Chailian Tang*
Source: *Yanke Zuanyao* (A Book Written by Huang Yan in 1867)
Radix Bupleuri
Rhizoma Coptidis
Radix Scutellariae
Radix Paeoniae Rubra
Fructus Viticis
Fructus Gardeniae
Radix Gentianae
Caulis Akebiae
Radix Glycyrrhizae
Herba Schizonepetae
Radix Ledebouriellae

40. *Longdan Xiegan Tang*
Source: *Lidong Hengfang* (Li Dong-heng's Recipe 1180-1251)
Radix Gentianae
Radix Bupleuri

Rhizoma Alismatis
Senem Plantaginis
Caulis Akebiae
Radix Rehmanniae
The Tip of Radix Angelicae Sinensis
Fructus Gardeniae
Radix Scutellariae
Radix Glycyrrhizae

41. *Tuoli Xiaodu San*
Source: *Yizong Jinjian* (The Golden Mirror of Medicine)
Radix Astragali seu Hedysari
Spina Gleditsiae
Flos Lonicerae
Radix Glycyrrhizae
Radix Platycodi
Radix Angelicae Dahuricae
Rhizoma Ligustici Chuanxiong
Radix Angelicae Sinensis
Radix Paeoniae Alba
Rhizoma Atractylodis Macrocephalae
Poria
Radix Ginseng

42. *Qianghuo Shengfeng Tang*
Source: *Yuanji Qiwei* (Revealing the Mystery of the Origin of Eye Diseases)
Radix Bupleuri
Herba Schizonepetae

Radix Ledebouriellae
Rhizoma seu Radix Notopterygii
Radix Angelicae Pubescentis
Herba Menthae
Rhizoma Ligustici Chuanxiong
Radix Angelicae Dahuricae
Rhizoma Atractylodis Macrocephalae
Radix Glycyrrhizae
Fructus Aurantii
Radix Scutellariae
Radix Platycodi
Radix Peucedani

43. *Zhi Bai Dihuang Tang*
Source: *Yizong Jinjian* (The Golden Mirror of Medicine)
Rhizoma Anemarrhenae
Cortex Phellodendri
Rhizoma Rehmanniae Praetaratae
Fructus Corni
Rhizoma Dioscoreae
Poria
Rhizoma Alismatis
Cortex Moutan Radicis

44. *Sang Ju Yi*
Source: *Wen Bin Tiao Bian* (Treatise on Differentiation and Treatment of Epidemic Febrile Diseases)
Folium Mori
Flos Chrysanthemi

Semen Armeniacae Amarum
Fructus Forsythiae
Radix Platycodi
Herba Menthae
Radix Glycyrrhizae
Rhizoma Phragmitis

45. *Yinhua Jiedu Tang*
Source: *Pangshi Jingyan Fang* (A book written by Dr. Pang)
Flos Lonicerae
Herba Taraxaci
Cortex Mori Radicis Praetarata
Radix Trichosanthis
Radix Scutellariae
Radix Gentianae
Radix et Rhizoma Rhei
Fructus Viticis
Fructus Aurantii

46. *Da Buyin Wan*
Source: *Dan Xi Xin Fa* (Danxi's Experiential Therapy)
Cortex Phellodendri (Parched with salt)
Rhizoma Anemarrhenae (Parched with salt)
Rhizoma Rehmanniae Praeparatae
Plastrum Testudinis

47. *Xiang Bei Yangrong Tang*
Source: *Yizong Jinjian* (A Golden Mirror of Medicine)
Rhizoma Atractylodis Macrocephalae

Radix Ginseng
Poria
Pericarpium Citri Reticulatae
Rhizoma Rehmanniae Praeparatae
Rhizoma Ligustici Chuanxiong
Radix Angelicae Sinensis
Bulbus Fritillariae
Rhizoma Cyperi
Radix Paeoniae Alba
Radix Platycodi
Radix Glycyrrhizae
Fructus Ziziphi Fujubae
Rhizoma Zingiberis Recens

48. *Shenling Baizhu San*
Source: *Heji Jufang* (A book written by Tai Ping Hui-ming in 1085)
Radix Codonopsis Pilosulae
Poria
Rhizoma Atractylodis Macrocephalae
Semen Dolichoris
Pericarpium Citri Retiulatae
Rhizoma Dioscoreae
Radix Glycyrrhizae Praeparata
Semen Nelumbinis
Semen Coicis
Radix Platycodi
Fructus Amomi Xanthioidis

49. Feier Wan
Source: *Yizong Jinjian* (A Golden Mirror of Medicine)
Radix Ginseng
Rhizoma Atractylodis Macrocephalae
Poria
Rhizoma Coptidis
Rhizoma Picrorhizae
Fructus Quisqualis
Massa Fermentata Medicinalis
Fructus Hordei Germinatus Praeparatae
Fructus Cratagaegi Praeparata
Radix Glycyrrhizae Praeparata
Aloe

50. Fuzi Lizhong Tang
Source: *Yanshi Xiaoer Fanglun* (A book written by Dr. Yan)
Radix Aconiti Praeparata
Rhizoma Atractylodis Macrocephalae
Rhizoma Zingiberis
Radix Codonopsis Pilosulae
Radix Glycyrrhizae Praeparata

51. Yiyang Jiulian San
Source: *Yuan Ji Qi Wei* (Revealing the Mystery of Origin of Eye Diseases)
Radix Rehmanniae
Radix Angelicae Pubescentis
Cortex Phellodendri
Radix Ledebouriellae

Rhizoma Anemarrhenae
Fructus Viticisp
Radix Peucedani
Rhizoma seu Radix Notopterygii
Radix Angelicae Dahuricae
Radix Glycyrrhizae
Radix Scutellariae
Calcitum
Fructus Gardeniae
Rhizoma Coptidis
Radix Stephaniae Tetrandrae

52. *Qiju Dihuang Tang*
Source: *Yizong Jinjian* (A Golden Mirror of Medicine)
Rhizoma Rehmanniae Praeparatae
Fructus Corni
Rhizoma Dioscoreae Praeparata
Rhizoma Alismatis
Poria
Cortex Moutan Radicis
Fructus Lycii
Flos Chrysanthemi

53. *Yiqi Congming Tang*
Source: *Pi Wei Lun* (Treatise on the Spleen and Stomach)
Fructus Viticis
Radix Astragali seu Hedysari
Radix Ginseng
Cortex Phellodendri

Radix Paeoniae Alba
Radix Glycyrrhizae Praeparata
Rhizoma Cimicifugae
Radix Puerariae

54. *Ganlu Yin*
Source: *Heji Jufang* (A book written by Tai Ping Hui-ming in 1085)
Radix Rehmanniae
Rhizoma Rehmanniae Praeparatae
Herba Dendrobii
Radix Asparagi
Radix Ophiopogonis
Radix Scutellariae
Herba Artemisiae Scopariae
Fructus Aurantii
Radix Glycyrrhizae
Folium Eriobotryae

55. *Chufeng Yisun Tang*
Source: *Shenshi Yaohan* (A Valuable Manual of Ophthalmology)
Radix Angelicae Sinensis
Radix Paeoniae Alba
Rhizoma Rehmanniae Praeparatae
Rhizoma Ligustici Chuanxiong
Rhizoma Ligustici
Radix Peucedani
Radix Ledebouriellae

56. *Mingmu Dihuang Tang*
Source: *Shenshi Yaohan* (A Valuable Manual of Ophthalmology)
Rhizoma Rehmanniae Preparatae
Fructus Corni
Rhizoma Dioscoreae Praeparata
Rhizoma Alismatis
Poria cum Ligno Hospitie
Radix Rehmanniae
Radix Bupleuri
Radix Angelicae Sinensis
Fructus Schisandrae
Cortex Moutan Radicis

57. *Dan Zhi Xiaoyao San*
Source: *Heji Jufeng* (A book written by Tai Ping Hui-ming in 1085)
Radix Bupleuri
Radix Angelicae Sinensis
Radix Paeoniae Alba
Poria
Rhizoma Atractylodis Macrocephalae
Radix Glycyrrhizae
Herba Menthae
Rhizoma Zingiberis Recens
Cortex Moutan Radicis
Fructus Gardeniae

58. *Lufeng Lingyang Yin*
Source: *Yizong Jinjian* (The Golden Mirror of Medicine)
Radix Scrophulariae
Radix Ledebouriellae
Poria
Rhizoma Anemarrhenae
Radix Scutellariae
Herba Asari
Radix Platycodi
Cornu Saigae Tataricae
Semen Plantaginis
Radix et Rhizoma Rhei

59. *Banxia Lingyangjiao San*
Source: *Shenshi Yaohan* (A Valuable manual of Ophthalmology)
Cornu Saigae Tataricae
Herba Menthae
Rhizoma seu Radix Notopterygii
Rhizoma Pinelliae
Flos Chrysanthemi
Radix Aconiti
Rhizoma Ligustici Chuanxiong
Radix Ledebouriellae
Senem Plantaginis
Herba Asari

60. *Lingyang Gouteng Yin*
Source: *Tongsu Shanghan Lun* (A book written by Yu

Gen-chu in Qing Dynasty)
Pulvis Cornu Saigae Tataricae
Ramulus Uncariae cum Uncis
Folium Mori
Flos Chrysanthemi
Radix Rehmanniae
Radix Paeoniae Alba
Radix Glycyrrhizae
Bulbus Fritillariae
Caulis Bambusae in Taeniam
Poria cum Ligno Hospite

61. *Lingyangjiao San*
Source: *Pu Ji Fang* (Prescriptions for Universal Relief)
Pulvis Cornu Saigae Tataricae
Poria cum Ligno Hospite
Semen Plantaginis
Flos Chrysanthemi
Semen Cassiae
Rhizoma seu Radix Notopterygii
Radix Ledebouriellae
Radix Paeoniae Rubra
Fructus Viticis
Radix Scutellariae
Rhizoma Cimicifugae
Fructus Gardeniae
Radix Ophiopogonis
Radix Glycyrrhizae
Radix Bupleuri

Fructus Aurantii

62. *Tongqiao Huoxie Tang*
Source: *Yi Lin Gai Cuo* (Corrections on the Errors of Medical Works)
Radix Paeoniae Rubra
Rhizoma Ligustici Chuanxiong
Semen Persicae
Flos Carthami
Fructus Ziziphi Jujubae
Rhizoma Zingiberis Recens
Allium Fistulosum
Moschus

63. *Di Tan Tang*
Source: *Jsheng Feng* (Prescriptions for Succouring the Sick)
Rhizoma Pinelliae
Exocarpium Citri Grandis
Poria
Radix Glycyrrhizae
Rhizoma Zingiberis Recens
Arisaema cum Bile
Fructus Aurantii Immaturus
Radix Ginseng
Acrous Calamus
Caulis Bambusae in Taeniam
Fructus Ziziphi Jujubae

64. *Tianma Gouteng Yin*

Source: *Zabing Zhengzhi Xinyi*
Rhizoma Gastrodiae
Ramulus Uncariae cum Uncis
Semen Cassiae
Fructus Gardeniae
Radix Scutellariae
Radix Cyathulae
Cortex Eucommiae
Herba Leonuri
Ramulus Loranthi
Caulis Polygoni Multiflori
Poria cum Ligno Hospite

65. *Jiajian Zhu Jing Wan*
Source: *Zongyi Yanke Liujimg Fayao* (A book written by Cheng Da-fu in 1971)
Semen Cuscutae
Fructus Broussonetiae
Fructus Leonuri
Fructus Lycii
Semen Plantaginis
Fructus Chaenomelis
Calcitum
Pulvis Placenta Hominis
Radix Notoginseng
Fructus Schisandrae

66. *Renshen Yangrong Tang*
Source: *Heji Jufang* (A book written by Tai Ping Hui-ming

in 1085)
Radix Ginseng
Poria
Rhizoma Atractylodis Macrocephalae
Radix Glycyrrhizae Praeparata
Radix Angelicae Sinensis
Rhizoma Rehmanniae Praeparatae
Radix Paeoniae Alba
Cortex Cinnamomi
Radix Astragali seu Hedysari
Radix Polygalae
Pericarpium Citri Reticulatae
Fructus Schisandrae
Rhizoma Zingiberis Recens
Fructus Ziziphi Jujubae

67. *Yougui Wan*
Source: *Jing Yue Quang Shu* (Complete Works of Zhang Jingyue)
Rhizoma Rehmanniae Praeparatae
Fructus Corni
Rhizoma Dioscoreae Praeparata
Fructus Lycii
Cortex Eucommiae
Radix Angelicae Sinensis
Cortex Cinnamomi
Radix Aconiti Praeparata
Semen Cuscutae
Colla Cornus Cervi

68. *Ba Zhen Tang*
Source: *Zheng Ti Lei Yao* (Classification and Treatment of Traumatic Diseases)
Radix Ginseng
Rhizoma Atractylodis Macrocephalae
Poria
Radix Angelicae Sinensis
Rhizoma Ligustici Chuanxiong
Radix Paeoniae Alba
Rhizoma Rehmanniae Praeparatae
Radix Glycyrrhizae

69. *Ning Xie Tang*
Source: (Experienced Recipe)
Herba Agrimoniae
Herba Ecliptae
Radix Rehmanniae
Fructus Gardeniae Carbonisetus
Radix Paeoniae Alba
Rhizoma Bletillae
Radix Ampelopsis
Cacumen Biotae
Colla Corii Asini
Rhizoma Imperatae

70. *Quyu Tang*
Source: *Zhongyi Yanke Xue* (Ophthalmology of TCM)
Rhizoma Ligustici Chuanxiong

the tip of Radix Angelicae Sinensis
Semen Persicae
Radix Paeoniae Rubra
Radix Rehmanniae
Herba Ecliptae
Herba Lycopi
Radix Salviae Miltiorrhizae
Herba Agrimoniae
Radix Curcumae

71. *Xianfang Huoming Yin*
Source: *Jiaozhu Furen Lianfang* (A book written by Cheng Zi-ming in Song Dynasty)
Radix Angelicae Dahuricae
Bulbus Fritillariae
Radix Ledebouriellae
Radix Paeoniae Rubra
the tip of Radix Angelicae Sinensis
Radix Glycyrrhizae
Spina Gleditsiae
Radix Trichosanthis
Resina Olibani
Resina Commiphorae Myrrhae
Flos Lonicerae
Pericarpium Citri Reticulatae
Squama Manitis

72. *Xienao Tang*
Source: *Shenshi Yaohan* (A Valuable Manual of

Ophthalmology)
Radix Ledebouriellae
Semen Plantaginis
Caulis Akebiae
Fructus Leonuri
Poria
Radix et Rhizoma Rhei
Radix Scrophulariae
Natrii Sulfas Exsiccatus
Radix Platycodi
Radix Scutellariae

73. *Tongyou Tang*
Source: *Lan Shimi Cang* (Secret Record of the Chamber of Orchids)
Radix Glycyrrhizae Praeparata
Flos Carthami
Radix Rehmanniae
Radix Rehmanniae Praeparatae
Rhizoma Cimicifugae
Semen Persicae
Radix Angelicae Sinensis

74. *Xiao Xuming Tang*
Source: *Qian Jin Fang* (Prescriptions Worth a Thousand Gold for Emergencies)
Herba Ephedrae
Radix Stephaniae Tetrandrae
Radix ginseng

Radix Scutellariae
Cortex Cinnamomi
Radix Glycyrrhizae
Radix Paeoniae
Rhizoma Ligustici Chuanxiong
Semen Armeniacae Amarum
Radix Aconiti Praeparata
Radix Ledebouriellae
Rhizoma Zingiberis Recens

75. *Liujunzi Tang*
Source: *Yi Xue Zheng Zhuang* (Orthodox Medical Problems)
Radix Ginseng
Rhizoma Atractylodis Macrocephalae
Poria
Radix Glycyrrhizae
Pericarpium Citri Reticulatae
Rhizoma Pinelliae
Rhizoma Zingiberis Recens
Fructus Ziziphi Jujubae

76. *Zheng Rong Tang*
Source: *Shenshi Yaohan* (A Valuable Manual of Ophthalmology)
Rhizoma seu Radix Notopterygii
Rhizoma Typhonii
Radix Ledebouriellae
Radix Gentianae Macrophyllae
Arisaema cum Bile

Bombyx Batryticatus
Rhizoma Pinellinae Praeparata
Fructus Chaenomelis
Lignum Pini Nodi
Radix Glycyrrhizae
Rhizoma Zingiberis Recens

77. *Buyang Huan Wu Tang*
Source: *Yi Lin Gai Cuo* (Corrections on the Errors of Medical Works)
Radix Astragali seu Hedysari
the tip of Radix Angelicae Sinensis
Radix Paeoniae Rubra
Lumbricus
Rhizoma Ligustici Chuanxiong
Semen Persicae
Flos Carthami

78. *Taohong Simu Tang*
Source: *Yizong Jinjian* (The Golden Mirror of Medicine)
Semen Persicae
Flos Carthami
Radix Angelicae Sinensis
Radix Rehmanniae
Radix Paeoniae Rubra
Rhizoma Ligustici Chuanxiong

79. *Tongxue Wan*
Source: *Zhengzhi Zhunsheng* (Standards of Diagnosis and

Treatment)
Radix Rehmanniae
Radix Paeoniae Rubra
Radix Glycyrrhizae
Rhizoma Ligustici Chuanxiong
Radix Ledebouriellae
Herba Schizonepetae
Radix Angelicae Sinensis

80. *Shihui San*
Source: *Shi Yao Shen Shu* (A Miraculous Book of Tan Prescriptions)
Herba seu Radix Cirsii Japonici
Herba Cephalanoploris
Folium Nelumbinis
Cacumen Biotae
Rhizoma Imperatae
Radix Rubiae
Fructus Gardeniae
Radix et Rhizoma Rhei
Cortex Moutan Radicis
Cortex Trachycarpi

81. *Xijiao Dihuang Tang*
Source: *Beiji Qianjin Yaofang* (Prescriptions Worth a Thousand Gold for Emergencies)
Cornu Rhinoceri
Radix Rehmanniae
Radix Paeoniae

Cortex Moutan Radicis

82. *Guipi Tang*
Source: *Ji Sheng Fang* (Prescriptions for Succouring the Sick)
Rhizoma Atractylodis Macrocephalae
Poria
Radix Astragali seu Hedysari
Radix Ginseng
Arillus Longan
Semen Ziziphi Spinosae
Radix Aucklandiae
Radix Glycyrrhizae
Radix Angelicae Sinensis
Radix Polygalae

83. *Xiaoyao San*
Source: *Heji Jufang* (A book written by Tai Ping Hui-ming in 1085)
Radix Bupleuri
Radix Angelicae Sinensis
Radix Paeoniae Albe
Rhizoma Atractylodis Macrocephalae
Poria
Radix Glycyrrhizae Praeparata
Herba Menthae
Rhizoma Zingiberis Recens

84. *Ruyi Jinhuang San*
Source: *Yizong Jinjian* (The Golden Mirror of Medicine)

Radix et Rhizoma Rhei	2.5 kg
Cortex Phellodendri	2.5 kg
Rhizoma Curcumae Longae	2.5 kg
Radix Angelicae Dahuricae	2.5 kg
Arisaema cum Bile	1 kg
Pericarpium Citri Reticulatae	1 kg
Rhizoma Atractylodis	1 kg
Cortex Magnoliae Officinalis	1 kg
Radix Glycyrrhizae	1 kg
Radix Trichosanthis	5 kg

All of the above are ground to very find powder.

85. *Fulan Kianyan Fang*

Source: *Shenshi Yaohan* (A Valuable Manual of Ophthalmology)

Calamina (Usta and Pulverisata)	30 g
Cinnabaris Pulverisata	15 g
Alumen Exsiccatum	7.5 g
Cinnabnris (grinded to be find powder)	3 g
Aerugo	6 g.

Mix the above together and grind to very fine powder

86. *Zijin Ding*

Source: *Pianyu Xinshu* (A book written by Ming Wan-quan in 1549)

Realgar
Cinnabaris
Moschus
Galla Chinensis

Radix Euphorbiae seu knoxiae (Moving away Aloe)
Bulbus Cremastrae (Clearing away peel and down)
Semen Euphorbiae Lathyridis Pulveratum

All are ground into very fine powder, using paste glutinous rice powder to make pastille. The weight of each partille is 0.03 g.

87. *Waizhang Yangyao Shui*
Source: *Jingyan Fang* (Experienced Prescriptions)

Rhizoma Coptidis	15 g
Natrii Sulfas Exsicatus	9 g
Borax	0.6 g
Stigma Croci	1.5 g.

Boil in water 1500g. for 30 minutes. Filter and add autiseptic.

88. *Huanglian Xigua Shuang Yanyi*
Source: *Jingyan Fang* (Experienced Prescriptions)

Berberine	0.5 g
Xigua Shuang	5.0 g
Borax	0.2 g
Nitrophenylmercuric	0.002 g.

Distilled water 100ml.

89. 100% *Qianli Guang Yanyao Shui*
Source: *Yiyuan Zhiji* (A book written by Ke Ming-qing, published in 1976)

Herba Senecionis Scandentis	10 g.

Immersed in alcohol, concentrated, decolorized, etc. Add distilled water till 100 ml. in the end.

90. *1% Huanglin Su Yanye*
Source: *Zhongyi Yanke Xue*
Baicalein Crystals   1 g.

Add distilled water 100 ml. and sodium hydroxide. Adjust pH to about 7. Then add 0.9% sodium chloride and 0.001% nitro-phenylmercuric as abtiseptic.

91. *Xihuang San*
Source: *Zhongyi Yanke Xue Jiangyi* (A book written by Gongdong Traditional Chinese Medical College in 1960)

Pulvis Borax Pulverisatus	15 g
Borneolum	9 g
Moschus	0.9 g
Caulculus Bovis	1.2 g.

(All are ground into very fine powder)

92. *Chunxue Gao*
Source: *Puji Fang* (Prescriptions for Universal Relief)

Borneolum	3 g
Nux Prinsepiae (Moving away shell)	6 g
Moschus	1.5 g.

(Grind into very fine powder and mix it with honey to make adhesive plaster.)

93. *Wudan Gao*
Source: *Yizong Jinjian* (The Golden Mirror of Medicine)
Pig Bile   7.5 g

Cattle Bile	7.5 g
Sheep Bile	7.5 g
Carp Blie	7.5 g
Fel Ursi	7.5 g
Pulvis Rhizoma Picrorhizae	7.5 g
Pulvis Rhizoma Coptidis	7.5 g
Pericarpium Citri Reticulatae Viride	7.5 g
Honey	60 g.

Mixed up with all of the above drugs, pour them into a china jar and seal it up. Steam them when cooking rice till the rice is done.

94. 10% *Huanglian Ye*
Source: *Yanke Linzheng Lu*

Radix Coptidis	10 g.

Boiled in water, filtered and make it up to 100ml. Add antiseptic and sterilized.

95. *Yinhuang Zhushe Ye*
Source: *Yiyuan Zhiji* (A book written by Ke Ming-qing, Published in 1960)

Extract of Flos Lonicerae	12.5 g
Extract of Radix Scutellariae	20 g
Benzyl alcohol	10 ml.
Water for injection	q.s

To make to 1000ml., filtered, preserved and sterilize.

96. 10% *Chuanxin Lianyan Ye*
Source: *Zhongyi Yanke Xue* (Ophthalmology of TCM)

Powder of extract of Herna Andrographitis   3 g

Add distilled water 100ml., adjust pH, and add antiseptic.

97. *Sanhuang Yanye*

Source: *Zhongyi Yanke Xue* (Ophthalmology of TCM)

Rhizoma Coptidis	6 g
Radix Scutellariae	6 g
Cortex Phellodendri	6 g.

Boiled in water twice, filtered, concentrated to 200ml., add Borax q.s., adjust pH, filtered and stirilized for use.

98. *Tuiyun San*

Source: *Yanke Linzheng Lu*

Bingxiang San	10 g
Calamina Praeparatae	60 g
To be group A	
Cortex Phellodendri	3 g
Radix Scutellariae	3 g
Rhizoma Coptidis	3 g
Radix Ledebouriellae	3 g
Periostracum Cicadae	3 g
Radix Angelicae Dahuricae	3 g
Rhizoma seu Radix Notopterygii	3 g
Herba Menthae	3 g
Rhizoma Ligustici Chuanxiong	3 g
Flos Chrysanthemi	3 g
Herba Schizonepetae	3 g
Radix Angelicae Sinensis	3 g
Radix et Rhizoma Rhei	3 g

Radix Paeoniae Rubra	3 g
Fructus Forsythiae	3 g
Herba Equiseti Hiemalis	3 g
To be group B	
Os Sepiellae seu Sepiae	6 g
Pulvis Cormus Eleocharis Dulcis	9 g
Borneolum Syntheticum	7.5 g
Calculus Boris	0.6 g
Pulvis Margarita	1.2 g
Fel Ursi	0.6 g
Sal–Ammoniaci	0.3 g
Cinnabaris	3 g.
Nux Prinsepiae	
Moschus	0.75 g
To be group C	

First, boil group B with water, filter, then add group A. Evaporate in the sun to make it dry. Grind it to very fine powder, then add group C. Grind it again to very fine powder and seal for use.

99. *Binglang Jiandi Yanye*
Source: *Zhongyi Yanke Xue* (Ophthalmology of TCM)

100. *Ding Gongteng Jian Diyanye*

101. *Lingqiao Jiedu Wan*
Source: *Quanguo Zhongcheng Yao Chufeng Ji*
Flos Lonicerae
Fructus Forsythiae

Radix Platycodi
Fructus Arctii
Herba Menthae
Herba Lophatheri
Spica Schizonepetae
Radix Glycyrrhizae
Semen Sojae Praeparatum
Cornu Antelopis

102. *Huanglian Shanqing Wan*
Source: *Quanguo Zhongcheng Yao Chufeng Ji*
Rhizoma Coptidis
Radix Scutellariae
Cortex Phellodendri
Fructus Gardeniae
Flos Chrysanthemi
Radix Angelicae Sinensis
Radix Platycodi
Radix Puerariae
Herba Menthae
Radix Scrophulariae
Radix Trichosanthis
Rhizoma Ligustici Chuanxiong
Rhizoma Curcumae Longae
Fructus Forsythiae
Radix et Rhizoma Rhei

103. *Niuhuang Jiedu Pian*
Source: *Youke Zhengzhi Zhunsheng* (A book written by

Wang Zhi-tang in 1607)
Calculus Bovis
Radix Glycyrrhizae
Flos Lonicerae
Rhizoma Bistortae

104. *Renshen Jianpi Wan*
Source: *Zabing Zhengzhi Neifeng* (A book written by Wang Zhi-tang in 1602)
Rhizoma Atractylodis Macrocephalae
Poria
Radix Ginseng
massa Fermentata Medicinalis
Pericarpium Citri Reticulata
Fructus Amomi
Fructus Hordei Germinatus
Fructus Crataegi
Rhizoma Dioscoreae
Semen Myristicae
Radix Aucklandiae
Rhizoma Coptidis
Radix Glycyrrhizae

105. *Shiquan Dabu Wan*
Source: *Heji Jufang* (A book written by Tai Ping Hui-ming in 1085)
Radix Ginseng
Rhizoma Atractylodis Macrocephalae
Radix Glycyrrhizae Praeparata

Radix Angelicae Sinensis
Rhizoma Ligustici Chuanxiong
Radix Paeoniae Alba
Radix Rehmanniae Praeparata
Radix Astragali seu Hedysari
Cortex Cinnamomi

106. *Niuhuang Qingxin Wan*
Source: *Douzhen Shiyi Xinfa* (Personal Insight of Smallpox and Rash Diseases)
Calculus Bovis
Cinnabaris
Fresh Rhizoma Coptidis
Radix Scutellariae
Fructus Gardeniae
Radix Curcumae

107. *Yangyin Qingfei Wan*
Source: *Quanguo Zhongcheng Yao Chufen Ji*
Radix Rehmanniae
Radix Scrophulariae
Bulbus Fritillariae Thunbergii
Herba Menthae
Radix Ophiopogonis
Cortex Moutan Radicis
Fresh Radix Paeoniae Alba
Radix Glycyrrhizae

108. *Liuwei Dihuang Wan*

Source: *Xiaoer Yaozheng Zhijue* (Key to Theraperutics of Children's Diseases)
Rhizoma Rehmanniae Praeparatae
Fructus Corni
Rhizoma Dioscoreae
Rhizoma Alismatis
Poria
Cortex Moutan Radicis

109. *Shihu Yeguang Wan*
Source: *Yuanji Qiwei* (Revealing the Mystery of the origin of Eye Diseases)
Radix Asparagi
Radix Ophiopogonis
Radix Ginseng
Poria
Rhizoma Rehmanniae Praeparatae
Rhizoma Rehmanniae
Radix Achyranthis Bidentatae
Semen Armeniacae Amarum
Fructus Lycii
Semen Cassiae
Rhizoma Ligustici Chuanxiong
Cornu Rhinoceri
Fructus Tribuli Alba
Cornu Antelopis
Fructus Aurantii
Herba dendrobii
Fructus Schisandrae

Semen Celosiae
Radix Glycyrrhizae
Radix Ledebouriellae
Herba Cistanchis
Rhizoma Coptidis
Flos Chrysanthemi
Rhizoma Dioscoreae
Semen Cuscutae

110. *Qiju Dihuang Wan:* The same as *Qiju Dihuang Tang*

111. *Xiaoyao Wan:* the same as *Xiaoyao San*

112. *Longdan Xiegan Wan:* The same as *Longdan Xiegan Tang*

113. *Zhibai Dihuang Wan:* The same as *Zhibai Dihuang Tang*

114. *Mingmu Dihuang Wan:* The same as *Mingmu Dihuang Tang*

115. *Buzhong Yiqi Wan:* The same as *Buzhong Yiqi Tang*

116. *Anshen Zhenjing Wan*
Source: *Ming Yi Za Zhu* (Collection of Experiences of Famous Physicians in the Ming Dynasty)
Concretion Silicea Bambusae
Radix Ginseng
Poria cum Ligno Hospite

Rhizoma Arisaematis Praeparata
Semen Ziziphi Spinosae (Fired)
Radix Angelicae Sinensis
Radix Rehmanniae
Radix Paeoniae Rubra
Herba Menthae
Caulis Akebiae
Rhizoma Coptidis
Fructus Gardeniae
Cinnabaris
Calculus Bovis
Os Draconis
Indigo Naturalis

17
眼 科 学

序

《英汉实用中医药大全》即将问世,吾为之高兴。

歧黄之道,历经沧桑,永盛不衰。吾中华民族之强盛,由之。世界医学之丰富和发展,亦由之。然而,世界民族之差异,国别之不同,语言之障碍,使中医中药的传播和交流受到了严重束缚。当前,世界各国人民学习、研究、运用中医药的热潮方兴未艾。为使吾中华民族优秀文化遗产之一的歧黄之道走向世界,光大其业,为世界人民造福,徐象才君集省内外精英于一堂,主持编译了《英汉实用中医药大全》。是书之问世将使海内外同道欢呼雀跃。

世界医学发展之日,当是歧黄之道光大之时。

吾欣然序之。

中华人民共和国卫生部副部长
　兼国家中医药管理局局长
世界针灸学会联合会主席
中国科学技术协会委员
中华全国中医学会副会长
中国针灸学会会长

胡熙明

1989年12月

序

中华民族有同疾病长期作斗争的光辉历程，故而有自己的传统医学——中国医药学。中国医药学有一套完整的从理论到实践的独特科学体系。几千年来，它不但被完好地保存下来，而且得到了发扬光大。它具有疗效显著、副作用小等优点，是人们防病治病，强身健体的有效工具。

任何一个国家在医学进步中所取得的成就，都是人类共同的财富，是没有国界的。医学成果的交流比任何其他科学成果的交流都应进行得更及时，更准确。我从事中医工作30多年来，一直盼望着有朝一日中国医药学能全面走向世界，为全人类解除病痛疾苦做出其应有的贡献。但由于用外语表达中医难度较大，中国医药学对外传播的速度一直不能令人满意。

山东中医学院的徐象才老师发起并主持了大型系列丛书《英汉实用中医药大全》的编译工作。这个工作是一项巨大工程，是一种大型科研活动，是一个大胆的尝试，是一件新事物。对徐象才老师及与其合作的全体编译者夜以继日地长期工作所付出的艰苦劳动，克服重重困难所表现出的坚韧不拔的毅力，以及因此而取得的重大成绩，我甚为敬佩。作为一个中医界的领导者，对他们的工作给予全力支持是我应尽的责任。

我相信《英汉实用中医药大全》无疑会在中国医学史和世界科学技术史上找到它应有的位置。

中华全国中医学会常务理事
山东省卫生厅副厅长

张奇文
1990年3月

出版前言

中国医药学是我中华民族优秀文化遗产之一，建国以来由于党和国家对待中医药采取了正确的政策，使中医药理论宝库不断得到了发掘整理，取得了巨大的成绩。当前，世界各国人民对中国医药学的学习和研究热潮日益高涨，为促进这一热潮更加蓬勃的发展，为使中国医药学能更好地为全人类解除病痛服务，就必须促进中医中药在世界范围内的传播和交流，而要使这一传播和交流进行得更及时、更准确，就必须首先排除语言障碍。因此，编译一套英汉对照的中医药基本知识的书籍，供国内外学习、研究中医药时使用，已成为国内外医药学界和医药学教育界许多人士的迫切需要。

多年来，在卫生部门的号召下，在"中医英语表达研究"方面，已经作出了一些可喜的成绩。本书《英汉实用中医药大全》的编辑出版就是在调查上述研究工作的历史和现状的基础上，继续对中医药英语表达作较系统、较全面的研究，以适应中国医药学对外传播交流的需要。

这部"大全"的版本为英汉对照，共有21个分册，一个分册介绍论述中国医药学的一个分科。在编著上注意了中医药汉文稿的编写特色，在内容上注意了科学性、实用性、全面性和简明易读。汉文稿的执笔撰写者主要是有20年以上实践经验的教授、副教授、主任医师和副主任医师。各分册汉文稿撰写成后，均经各学科专家逐一审订。各分册英文主译、主审主要是国内既懂中医又懂英语的权威人士，还有许多中医院校的英语教师及医药卫生部门的专业翻译人员。英译稿脱稿后，经过了复审、终审，有些译稿还召开全国22所院校和单位人员参加的英译稿统稿定稿研讨会，对英译稿进行细致的研讨和推敲，对如何较全面、较系统、较准确地用英语表达中国医药学进行了探讨，从而推动整个译文达到较高水平，因此，这部"大全"可供中医院校高年级学生作为泛读教材使用。

这部"大全"的编纂得到了国家教育委员会、国家中医药管理局、山东省教育委员会、山东省卫生厅等各部门有关领导的支持。在国家教委高等教育司的指导下，成立了《英汉实用中医药大全》编译领导委员会。还得到了全国许多中医院校和中药生产厂家领导的支持。

希望这部"大全"的出版，对中医院校加强中医英语教学，对国内卫生界培养外向型中医药人才，以及在推动世界各国人民对中医药的学习和研究方面，都将产生良好的影响。

高等教育出版社
1990年3月

前　言

《英汉实用中医药大全》是一部以中医基本理论为基础，以中医临床为重点，较为全面系统、简明扼要、易读实用的中级英汉学术性著作。它的主要读者是：中医药院校高年级学生和中青年教师，中医院的中青年医生和中医药科研单位的科研人员，从事中医对外函授工作的人员和出国讲学或行医的中医人员，西学中人员，来华学习中医的外国留学生和各类进修人员。

由于中国医药学为我中华民族之独有，因此，英译便成了本《大全》编译工作的重点。为确保译文能准确表达中医的确切含义，我们邀集熟悉中医的英语人员、医学专业翻译人员、懂英语的中医药人员乃至医古文人员于一堂，共同翻译、共同对译文进行研讨推敲的集体翻译法，这样，就把众人之长融进了译文质量之中。然而，即使这样，也难确保译文都能尽如人意。汉文稿虽反映了中国医药学的精髓和概貌，但也难能十全十美。我衷心地盼望读者能提出批评和建议，以便《大全》再版时修改。

参加本《大全》编、译、审工作的人员达200余名，他们来自全国28个单位，其中有山东、北京、上海、天津、南京、浙江、安徽、河南、湖北、广西、贵阳、甘肃、成都、山西、长春等15所中医学院，还有中国中医研究院，山东省中医药研究所等中医药科研单位。

山东省教育委员会把本《大全》的编译列入了科研计划并拨发了科研经费，山东省卫生厅和一些中药生产厂家也给了很大支持，济南中药厂的资助为编译工作的开端提供了条件。

本《大全》的编译成功是全体编译审者集体劳动的结晶，是各有关单位主管领导支持的结果。在《大全》各分册即将陆续出版之际，我诚挚地感谢全体编译审者的真诚合作，感谢许多专家、教授、各级领导和生产厂家的热情支持。

愿本《大全》的出版能在培养通晓英语的中医人才和使中医早日全面走向世界方面起到我所期望的作用。

主编　徐象才

于山东中医学院

1990年3月

目 录

说明 …………………………………………………………… 282
1 眼与脏腑经络的关系 ………………………………………… 283
　1.1 眼与脏腑的关系 ………………………………………… 283
　1.2 眼与经络的关系 ………………………………………… 285
　1.3 五轮学说及其应用 ……………………………………… 286
2 病因病机 ……………………………………………………… 288
　2.1 病因 ……………………………………………………… 288
　2.2 病机 ……………………………………………………… 291
3 眼科常用辨证法 ……………………………………………… 294
　3.1 辨外障及内障 …………………………………………… 294
　3.2 常见症状辨证 …………………………………………… 294
　3.3 辨眼底常见症 …………………………………………… 295
4 治疗概要 ……………………………………………………… 297
　4.1 内治法 …………………………………………………… 297
　4.2 外治法 …………………………………………………… 301
　4.3 眼科常用药物 …………………………………………… 304
5 眼睑疾病 ……………………………………………………… 311
　5.1 麦粒肿 …………………………………………………… 311
　5.2 眼睑脓肿 ………………………………………………… 313
　5.3 眼睑丹毒 ………………………………………………… 314
　5.4 眼睑湿疹 ………………………………………………… 316
　5.5 霰粒肿 …………………………………………………… 317
　5.6 睑缘炎 …………………………………………………… 318
　5.7 上睑下垂 ………………………………………………… 320

6 泪器疾病 … 323
- 6.1 泪道功能不全 … 323
- 6.2 慢性泪囊炎 … 324
- 6.3 急性泪囊炎 … 326

7 结膜疾病 … 328
- 7.1 沙眼 … 328
- 7.2 急性卡他性结膜炎 … 330
- 7.3 流行性急性结膜炎 … 332
- 7.4 慢性卡他性结膜炎 … 333
- 7.5 泡性结膜炎 … 334
- 7.6 春季卡他性结膜炎 … 336
- 7.7 翼状胬肉 … 337

8 巩膜疾病 … 339
- 8.1 巩膜炎 … 339

9 角膜疾病 … 341
- 9.1 匐行性角膜溃疡 … 341
- 9.2 单纯疱疹性角膜炎 … 343
- 9.3 深层角膜炎 … 345
- 9.4 束状角膜炎 … 346
- 9.5 角膜软化症 … 347

10 色素膜疾病 … 350
- 10.1 急性渗出性虹膜睫状体炎 … 350
- 10.2 慢性色素膜炎 … 351

11 晶状体疾病 … 353
- 11.1 老年性白内障 … 353
- 11.2 外伤性白内障 … 355

12 青光眼 … 357
- 12.1 急性闭角型青光眼 … 357
- 12.2 开角型青光眼 … 359

13　眼底疾病 …………………………………………… 361
13.1　视网膜中央血管阻塞 ………………………… 361
13.2　视网膜静脉周围炎 …………………………… 363
13.3　中心性浆液性脉络膜视网膜病变 …………… 365
13.4　视网膜色素变性 ……………………………… 367
13.5　视神经炎 ……………………………………… 369

14　玻璃体疾病 ………………………………………… 372
14.1　玻璃体混浊 …………………………………… 372

15　眼眶疾病 …………………………………………… 374
15.1　眼眶急性炎症 ………………………………… 374
15.2　眼眶假性肿瘤 ………………………………… 375

16　眼肌疾病 …………………………………………… 377
16.1　麻痹性斜视 …………………………………… 377
16.2　共同性斜视 …………………………………… 378

17　眼外伤 ……………………………………………… 380
17.1　眼挫伤 ………………………………………… 380
17.2　眼球穿通伤 …………………………………… 381

附篇 ……………………………………………………… 384

英汉实用中医药大全(书目) …………………………… 399

说　　明

　　眼科学是《英汉实用中医药大全》的第 17 分册。

　　本分册共有 17 章和附篇。1 至 4 章简明扼要地介绍了中医眼科的基础理论；5 至 17 章介绍了用中医药治疗 41 种常见眼病的诊治方法。对每种眼病都用现代医学病名表示，并从病因病机、临床表现、辨证论治 3 个方面对其进行阐述。在治疗时采用了"同病异治"，"异病同治"，辨病与辨证相结合的方法。附篇介绍了中医眼科常用方剂。

　　本分册汉文稿由南京中医学院陆绵绵教授审阅。

编者

1 眼与脏腑经络的关系

人体是一个有机的整体，各个组织器官之间，不论是生理功能，还是病理变化，都有着不可分割的关系，相互联系，互相影响。眼睛是人体的视觉器官，是机体的一个重要组成部分，因此，它与机体的脏腑器官、经络、气血等都保持着密切的联系。如果脏腑、经络、气血功能失调，即可反映于眼部，进而导致眼病。反之，眼部疾病也可通过经络、气血影响脏腑，使之功能失调而引起全身性反应。所以，在研究眼病的病因病机及辨证施治时，不能孤立地只看局部，必须从整体观念出发，联系眼与脏腑、经络之间的关系，进行全面观察和综合分析。

1.1 眼与脏腑的关系

眼之所以能视万物，辨别颜色，全赖五脏六腑精气的濡养，故曰五脏六腑之精气皆上注于目而为之精，精即指视觉功能。若脏腑功能失调，精气不能输注于目，就会影响眼的视功能，导致眼病。

肝，开窍于目。肝受血而能视。肝气通于目，肝和则目能辨五色。肝主藏血，具有贮藏血液调节血量的功能。肝主疏泄，具有调畅人体气机的功能。肝血充足，肝气条达舒畅，则所藏的精微物质在气的推动鼓舞下，源源不断地输送至眼，使眼得到滋养，从而维持正常的视觉功能。若肝血不足，肝阴亏虚，或肝气虚不能输送精微物质上注于目，致使眼失所养，则导致目昏眼花，视物不清。若肝气郁结，则气机不利，肝失疏泄其气上逆，血随其上，致使气滞血淤或血溢脉外，均能导致眼病。肝与胆互为表里，脏腑相合，肝之余气溢于胆，聚集成精则为胆汁。胆汁渗润升发于目，积聚而成神膏(玻璃体)、神水(房水)，濡养瞳神则视物清晰。若胆热内盛，灼煎神膏、神水，使之混浊不清，瞳神失养则视物不明。

诸血者，皆属于心。诸脉者，皆属于目。心脏主管全身血脉，脉中血液受心气推动，循环全身，上输于目，眼受血养，方能维持正常视觉，即目得血而能视。若心火内盛，灼伤脉络则血溢脉外，或致血脉淤阻，使气血供给中断，目失滋养则视力下降，甚至失明。心气充足，功能正常，则人体精神焕发，眼睛炯炯有神，活动灵活。心气虚或阴血不足，则心主血脉的功能失常，血液不能上注于目，则视物昏暗，神疲而目无神，故目为心之使，又为心之外窍。心与小肠相表里，脏腑相合。小肠有分别浊的功能，所谓清，包括津液和水谷之精气，由小肠吸收且输转于脾，再由脾输布上注于目，因此眼睛湿润有光泽，活动灵活，视物清楚。若小肠分清别浊功能失职，则眼失滋养而干涩不适，视物模糊不清。

肾者主水，受五脏六腑之精而藏之。眼睛的视功能要依赖于五脏六腑精气的濡养，而肾为藏精之所，所以视觉是否正常，与肾所藏精气的多少有密切关系。虽然肝开窍于目，但肾却司其明，只有肾气正常，肾精充足，上充满目，眼才能发挥其视觉功能。若肾脏虚损，藏精不足，则目眈眈无所见。肾藏精，精生髓，脑为髓之海，眼与脑通过目系相联，故肾虚则髓海不足，致目无所见。肾脏有气化水液的功能，对人体内部水液的分布、潴留、排泄具有特别重要的意义。气化功能正常，则将水分津液化为泪液、神水，以润泽、滋养眼球。气化功能失职，则造成水湿内停，上犯于目，则视物不清，视物变形。肾与膀胱相表里，脏腑相合。膀胱具有气化行水、排泄尿液的功能。膀胱气化功能正常，则清气上充于目，浊气下排体外，目明而亮。气化失常，清浊不分，水湿内停久则化热，湿热蒸腾于目，则视物如雾中行，曚昧不清，或眼前黑影飘浮。

五脏之气，上通九窍。五脏禀受气于六腑，六腑受气于胃。五脏六腑之精气，皆禀受于脾，上贯于目。所以，眼与脾胃关系十分密切。脾主运化升清，胃主降浊。脾胃功能正常，则清阳之精气上贯于目，目得濡养而能辨细微。眼肌受养，则眼球运动自如，开合灵活。反之，清阳不升，目失所养，浊阴不降，上泛于目，则目疾生矣。脾统血，血养目，由于脾的统摄作用，使血液行于眼的脉络之中而不外溢，以达养目之目的。脾虚统摄无权，便引起眼部出血疾病。

肺主宣发，能使气血津液敷布于目，肺又主肃降，能使水液运行下输膀胱。肺的宣降功能正常，则血脉通利，目得温养，能卫外抗邪而目不病。若宣降失常，气机不利，气滞血淤会致目疾。肺与大肠互为表里，脏腑相合，功能互相影响。若大肠积热，腑气不通，可使肺气不降，也会导致眼病。若肺失肃降，则腑气推动无力，可致大肠不畅，久则积热，阳明热盛，亦可致眼病。

1.2 眼与经络的关系

12经脉，365络，其血气皆上头面而走空窍，其精阳气上走于目而为精。经络有连络脏腑，沟通表里，运行气血的作用。五脏六腑之精气，亦靠经络的运行而上注于目。眼与经络的联系，可归纳为3种形式：一是直接通于目，如足厥阴肝经连目系，足少阳胆经起于目锐眦，足太阳膀胱经起于目内眦，足阳明胃经入目内眦。二是支络连于目，如手少阴心经支络连于目系，手太阳小肠经、手少阳三焦经支络入目锐眦。三是其他经络通过别络与眼有联系。在病理上，外感六淫，内伤七情，都可通过经络，从眼部影响脏腑，或从脏腑影响眼部。

1.3　五轮学说及其应用

五轮学说的理论是以《内经》为基础。《内经》中指出眼的各部分与脏腑的关系，为五轮学说的建立奠定了基础。五轮学说将眼由外向内，分为肉轮、血轮、气轮、风轮、水轮5部分，并分属五脏，借以说明眼的解剖、生理、病理与脏腑的关系。随着脏腑学说的发展、充实和完善，五轮学说的内容亦更加丰富，理论也更加完善。至今仍广泛的应用于临床辨证治疗。

肉轮，指胞睑，即眼睑，包括眼睑皮肤、皮下组织、肌肉、睑板、睑结膜等。它是眼睛的最外部分，其功能司开合，在脏属脾，脾主肌肉，故称肉轮。脾胃相表里，脾胃功能正常，则眼睑色泽正常，开合自如。若脾虚，中气不足，眼睑失养，则松弛无力，抬举困难。睑弦红赤湿烂，多属脾胃湿热蒸腾。胃火炽盛，阳明腑实，则眼睑红肿疼痛。

血轮，指两眦，包括两眦部的皮肤、内眦部的半月皱襞、泪阜、泪小点、泪道、泪囊及两眦部的部分球结膜、巩膜。两眦在脏属心，心主血，故称血轮。心功能正常，心血畅旺，则眦部皮肤荣润光泽。若心火上炎，可使泪窍红赤疼痛。

气轮，指白睛，即球结膜、巩膜。在脏属肺，肺主气，故称气轮。巩膜质地坚韧，具有保护眼内组织的作用。肺气充足，卫外固摄，邪不可入。肺阴充沛，白睛色白而润泽。肺阴不足，则白睛干燥无光泽。

风轮，指黑睛，即角膜，质地坚韧、光泽透明，与巩膜相连形成眼球的最外层。在脏属肝，肝主风，故称风轮。肝气调达，肝阴充足，则黑睛清莹，表面光滑，视物清晰。若肝经有火热之邪，上犯于目，则黑睛生翳，混浊不清，视物模糊。

水轮，指瞳神，包括房水、虹膜、瞳孔、晶状体、玻璃体、视网膜、视神经、脉络膜。瞳神在脏属肾，肾主水，故称水轮，是视物的重要部分。肾精充足，目得滋养，则瞳神清莹明沏，展缩灵活，视物清楚。肾精不足，津液亏损，则瞳神暗淡，甚而变白。

总之，五轮学说明确了眼各个部位与脏腑的具体联系、即轮脏隶属关系。在临床上，有时可以根据眼某部的证候，以推断某脏的病变。

(伊成运)

2 病因病机

2.1 病因

病因是指引起人体发生疾病的原因。眼直接与外界环境接触，同时与脏腑经络又有密切的联系，因此很容易受体内外因素的影响而发病。中医眼病的病因学说，既重视内外致病因素即邪气，也十分重视机体抗病因素即正气。即邪之所凑，其气必虚。眼病的发生、转归，是正邪斗争的反映。眼病的病因，可分为外因、内因、不内外因。外因，即指风、寒、暑、湿、燥、火六淫及疠气，但六淫之中，眼最易遭受风火外邪侵袭。内因，即指喜、怒、忧、思、悲、恐、惊七情，情志过极，七情内移，脏腑功能紊乱，气血失调而致眼病。不内外因，包括外伤、饮食不节、劳累过度等。

六淫

风、寒、暑、湿、燥、火，正常状态下称六气，在太过、不及、或非应时而至引起眼病的情况下称六淫。六淫之邪可以乘机侵袭肌表、口鼻，由表入里，或循经上犯引起眼病；也可以直接侵袭眼部而发病。可以单独致病，也可以兼挟为害，具有明显的季节性，以外障眼病多见。

风：风为阳邪，具有向上、向外、升发的特性。古人云："伤于风者，上先受之"。眼居体表、上部，所以最易受风邪侵扰而致病，特别以胞睑、眦部、白睛、黑睛病多见。风为六淫中首要的致病因素，除单独引起眼病外，还常为其他外邪入侵的先导，挟寒、湿、燥、火上犯于目致病。风者喜行而数变。故由风邪引起的眼病，发病突然，变化迅速。如风邪侵袭引起的暴风客热、黑睛生翳、红肿赤痛多猝然发病。风邪致病在眼部的主要表现有：目痒、目涩、羞明、流泪、目赤、黑睛生翳、胞睑浮肿、上睑下垂、风牵偏视等。

火：火为阳邪，其性上炎，故易于犯目而发病，其它外邪侵袭机体，亦易从火化。火本是人体生命的原动力，得其正即为阳气，失其正则为邪热，热为火之渐，火为热之甚，因此，火热难以截然分开。火为阳，因阳主升，火热同性，皆升腾炎上，最易上冲头目致病。火热之邪多引起眼睑红肿疼痛，生疮溃脓。火热致病在眼部的主要表现有：怕热羞明、涩痛难睁、目赤、灼热刺痒、热泪如汤、眵多黄稠、眼睑红赤、胀痛拒按、白睛赤肿溢血、黑睛生翳溃陷或突起等症。多致黄液上冲、瞳神紧小、暴盲、血灌瞳神等病。

湿：其性重浊粘腻，滞而不行，为阴邪。阳气易受其困扰而升发功能不得发越，所以湿邪致病，起病常较缓慢，病程缠绵，时好时坏，难于短期治愈。湿邪侵入机体，依患者阳气盛衰情况可化热生寒，导致湿热内蕴或寒湿内停。湿邪致病在眼部的临床表现有：眵泪胶粘、睑弦赤烂、湿痒起水泡、水泡溃后流黄水结痂、白睛黄赤或污红、视物模糊、视网膜水肿或渗出。

寒：寒为阴邪，其性凝滞。寒邪外袭，易伤阳气，阳气亏虚则目失温养，可致冷泪时流，视物昏花。寒邪侵袭，滞留于眼睑皮肉血脉之间，致气滞血凝，证见眼睑紫胀、白睛脉络紫滞或色淡红。寒邪侵袭，伤及经络，可见眼睑紧涩不适。

燥：燥为阳邪，其性干涩，极易耗伤津液。燥邪致病，在眼部的主要表现为：眼睛干涩不适、频频眨目、眼眵干结、白睛红赤、少津无光泽、甚见皱褶、久则黑睛混浊失去光泽、视物不清。

暑：暑为阳邪，其性炎热，极易伤津耗液。暑邪常挟湿致病，症见目赤肿痛、视物昏矇不明、眼睑湿疹水泡、糜烂溃疡等。

至於内风、内火、内寒、内湿、内燥之邪，是由于脏腑、气血、津液功能失调或紊乱所产生的，其所致眼病的表现将在下一节涉及。

六淫之中，一种邪气单独致病者较少，多种邪气相兼致病较多，其中以风热、风火多见。人是一个有机整体，眼与全身有着密切的联系，所以六淫致病不仅有眼局部的表现，并伴有一些全身症状。同样，由六淫所致的全身性疾病，也常常出现某些眼部症状，或合并某些眼病。因此，在眼科临床辨证时，必须将局部和整体的症状结合起来分析。

疠气

疠气是具有强烈传染性的致病邪气，眼科所见致病的疠气，性多温热。感邪之后，其特点是发病突然，来势凶猛，变化迅速，传染性很强，常引起广泛性流行。其临床表现，多见白睛红赤水肿、眼睑浮肿、热泪频流、羞明怕热、甚而黑睛生翳、眼球疼痛。

七情

在正常情况下，情志变化是正常的精神活动表现，脏腑精气为其物质基础。若七情变化过度，则影响脏腑正常生理功能，使气机升降失常，功能紊乱，精气不能上注于目，引起眼部疾病或全身性疾病的眼部症状。情志过度，往往导致气行失常，一般以气结闭塞较为常见，气结又可化火上炎。情志内伤所致眼部症状表现各异，常见的有：冷泪常流、酸涩微赤、目珠胀痛、视物不清、黑睛生翳、暴盲、青盲、五风内障等。

饮食不节

饮食为人体摄取营养，维持生命活动所必须的物质。若食无规律，饥饱无度，可以损害脾胃的正常功能，脾胃为后天之本，脏腑精气皆禀受于脾胃而上贯于目。食少则气血生化之源缺乏，久则脏腑精气衰竭；过量则损伤脾胃，致运化功能失常，营血精气无以化生，故精气亏虚不能濡目而引起眼病。如上睑下垂、视瞻昏渺、青盲等。若过食膏粱厚味，辛辣炙煿之品，尤其饮酒过度，常致脾胃内蕴湿热痰浊，上乘眼部则表现为：眼睑肿痛、赤烂、痰核、疮疡等。湿浊上犯于目，则引起视物昏花，视网膜水肿、渗出、出血。小儿偏食，久则气虚血少，目失濡养，可致雀目、疳积上目。

劳倦

劳倦主要是指过用体力、脑力、目力、房事过度，致使营血亏虚，阴精暗耗。一则目失滋养，二则虚火上乘，均可引起眼病，如青盲，视瞻昏渺、圆翳内障等。

2.2 病机

病机是指疾病发生、发展及变化的机理。讨论眼病的病机，不能离开整体观念，当致病因素引起人体阴阳失去相对平衡，气机升降失调，脏腑、经络、气血功能紊乱时，就能导致眼病。由于人机体的体质各异，病因繁多，所以导致眼病的病机也很复杂。

脏腑功能失调

肝胆功能失调：临床上，由肝胆功能失调所致的眼病以实证居多，且多为火邪或湿热熏蒸上犯。虚证多属肝阴亏损、肝血不足。虚实兼杂者，则以阴虚火旺、肝风内动多见。肝胆实火，肝郁化火或邪传少阳、厥阴之经，气火上逆，攻冲头目，风轮受损，则目赤肿痛、羞明热泪、黑睛生翳、溃陷、瞳神紧小。若热入血分，灼伤目中血络，迫血妄行可致眼内出血。肝郁气滞，肝失疏泄，气机郁滞，经脉不利，气血津液滞而不行，可致目赤视昏；甚而眼球胀痛坚硬，牵连头额，视力下降。气滞血瘀，筋脉失养，可致眼球转动疼，视物不清及暴盲。肝胆湿热，湿热内蕴，蒸腾于上，浊气上泛，上壅头目，则头目不利，白睛红赤秽浊，黑睛生翳如凝脂。肝血不足，肝藏血，目得血而能视，肝虚血少，目失濡养则眼干涩不适，视物模糊，甚而盲无所见。若小儿肝虚血少，则致夜盲，进而白睛黑睛干燥无光泽。肝阴亏虚，不能制约肝阳，阳亢于上，可引起眼疼，目红赤而视物不清。肝阴亏损，虚火上炎，肝风内动，风火相助，上攻头目，可致头痛眼胀，眼球偏斜，眼睑振跳。

肾膀胱功能失调：肾与膀胱功能失调所引起的眼病属实证者少，多属虚，主要有肾阴虚、肾阳虚。肝肾同源，肝肾阴虚，阴精不能上濡头目，可致睛珠混浊，眼球隐痛，眼球转动时牵拉样痛，视力下降，头晕目眩。肾阳虚衰，温煦生化功能不足，目失温养，可致目暗不明。阳虚火衰，不能温化水液，使水液内停，上泛溢于眼睑肌肤之间，则眼睑浮肿，溢于眼内则见视网膜水肿、渗出、甚而视网膜脱离。若热结膀胱则气化失职，湿热熏蒸，可致目赤头痛，白睛晦暗。

心与小肠功能失调：心与小肠功能失调引起的眼病，实证多属心火亢盛，虚证多为心阴亏虚。心火亢盛，上炎于目，燔灼血络，热入血分，可致眼球针刺样疼痛，内眦部白睛红赤，脉络粗大，胬肉肥厚，甚而血热壅盛，血溢脉外，致使白睛溢血，眼内出血，视力下降。火毒内盛，还可引起眼生疮疡，肉腐成脓。阴亏血虚，目失所养，则眼干涩痒，视物不清。虚火上炎，则白睛淡红，羞明流泪。

脾胃功能失调：脾胃功能失调所致眼病，病机多属胃火炽盛、脾胃湿热、脾虚气弱、脾不统血。胃火炽盛，火邪循经上炎于目，使局部气血淤阻，脉络不通，可引起球结膜充血、水肿，眼睑肿胀而硬，甚而引起眼睑脓肿。阳明热盛，热毒上攻，虹膜受灼，还可致房水混浊，瞳孔缩小。脾胃湿热，湿热熏蒸，浊气上泛，蒙蔽清窍，可致视网膜水肿、渗出、出血，视物不清。湿热停滞于眼睑，气血运行不畅，可致乳头肥大，滤泡增生，睑缘见细小水泡，红赤湿烂结痂，甚而眼睑红肿疼痛，生疮溃脓。湿热困脾，脾阳不振，运化失职，致使痰湿内聚，阻塞眼睑脉络，可致眼睑重坠浮肿，久则积聚成块。脾虚气弱，精血生化不足，眼睑筋脉肌肉失养，则眼睑松弛，下垂不能抬举。脾不统血，可使目中血不循经而溢于络外，轻则视物不清，眼前黑影飘移，重则视物不见。

肺与大肠功能失调：肺大肠功能失调所致眼病，实证多由外邪犯肺，肺失宣降所致，虚证多属肺阴不足。风热袭肺，肺失宣降，则致肺的敷布功能失常，气血阻滞目中脉络，则球结膜充血，血管粗大迂曲，水液不能下输膀胱而上壅于目，则致眼球胀痛，球结膜水肿。肺热内盛，上炎于目，则眼怕热羞明，眵多粘稠，球结膜充血水肿，甚而巩膜充血紫暗。热入血分，迫血妄行，灼伤脉络，可致球结膜出血。肺阴不足，虚火上炎，目失润养，可致眼干涩隐痛，眼眵干结，球结膜充血久而不退。

气血功能失调

气虚气陷：正气亏虚，阳气不能升散，致目失荣养，卫外不固，统摄、温煦失职，在眼部主要表现为上睑下垂、冷泪常流、角膜溃陷久不平复愈合、视疲劳等。

气滞气逆：气机阻塞，运行不畅，升降失常，均可致眼病。肺气不宣，阻滞脉络，可致球结膜充血，结节样隆起。肝气郁滞，可上逆化火，气火上逆，血随其上，火灼脉络则血溢脉外，可致眼球胀痛、视物昏花、眼底出血及眼球转动时隐痛。

血热：血得热则畅流，见眼部红肿热痛，血受热迫，灼伤脉络，血溢脉外，可见球结膜出血、眼内出血。

血瘀：眼部血行淤滞，可见眼睑紫暗，球结膜、巩膜充血紫暗血管粗大，视网膜阻滞可见视网膜水肿、出血、视力下降，疼痛剧烈，痛有定处，持续不解。

血虚：血虚不能上荣头目，则见头晕目眩，视物昏花，眼睑色淡，眼干涩不能久视，干燥无光泽，眼球隐痛，目痒时作。

(伊成运)

3 眼科常用辨证法

眼科辨证方法与内科相似,但也有独特之处,一般急性眼病多以局部辨证为主,慢性眼病多以全身辨证为主。现介绍几种常用局部辨证。

3.1 辨外障及内障

外障:指眼球表面及附属器的疾病。外障多为外感六淫,亦可由痰湿内聚、脾气虚弱、肝肾不足、外伤等因素致病。其特点是起病急,发展快,外部症状明显,如眼睑红肿,球结膜充血,角膜混浊,畏光,流泪等。一般来说,急性的外障为实证,慢性的外障多为虚证。

内障:指眼球内部各组织及视神经的疾病。内障多由七情内伤、劳倦、外伤等因素致脏腑、经络、气血功能失调所致。内障以视功能障碍为主,外眼多正常。内障多为虚证,也可虚实相兼。

3.2 常见症状辨证

辨视觉:视力减退伴睫状充血或混合性充血,多为外感风热或肝胆火炽;视力缓降,眼前有黑影飘动,或视物变形,外观正常,多为痰湿内困、肝肾不足、气血两亏;外眼正常,视力骤降,多为气血淤闭、血热妄行、肝胆火盛、阴虚火旺。

辨红肿:眼睑红肿痛为脾胃热毒蕴积;眼睑浮肿,但不红不痛为脾肾阳虚,水湿上犯;睑红肿皮肤湿烂为湿热蕴积;睑皮肤青紫为血淤。

球结膜充血、流泪、分泌物多为外感风热,或肺经实热;球结膜水肿，无充血为肺气不利；睫状充血或混合性充血为肝胆实热；局限性充血为肺经积热肺气不宣。

辨痛痒：一般暴痛为实症，久痛为虚症。痛而拒按喜冷为实热；痛而喜按畏冷为虚寒；日间痛属阳，夜间痛属阴；剧痛或胀痛为肝胆火炽；隐痛为阴虚火旺。

目痒多属风，有虚实之分；目痒也可由食物或药物过敏引起。目痒难忍兼流泪、球结膜充血为风热外袭；痒而睑皮肤红肿湿烂为脾胃湿热，复感风邪；目病将愈而痒为气血得行，脉络通畅；目微痒时作时止为血虚生风。

辨眵泪：眵多而稠黄为热毒炽盛；眵多硬结为肺经实热；眵稀不结为肺经虚热；眵泪胶粘为湿热壅盛。

泪液有冷热之分，泪多而热为风热毒邪或外伤；迎风流泪或冷泪长流为肝肾不足。

辨翳膜：指角膜疾病而言。新翳为炎症性混浊，初起翳如星状，树枝状为肝经风热；若形成溃疡或合并虹膜炎为热毒壅盛；溃疡日久不愈为正虚邪留。角膜炎症痊愈，遗留瘢痕混浊称老翳，又称宿翳。

膜系指从角膜缘向中央蔓延之膜。膜有大量新生血管或呈肉样称赤膜，多为肝肺风热炽盛，脉络淤滞；膜菲薄不充血称白膜，多为肺气盛。

3.3 辨眼底常见症

视神经乳头：视神经乳头充血水肿、边界模糊为肝经风热或肝郁气滞；视神经乳头苍白，动脉细为肝血不足或气血两亏；视神经乳头水肿为气血郁滞或脾肾阳虚。

视网膜血管：视网膜动脉变细多为肝阳上亢，或肝风内动；视网膜动脉呈白线状多为风痰阻络；或肝风内动；动静脉均细为气血不足；视网膜静脉扩张迂曲为气滞血淤，或心火上炎，或阴虚火旺。

黄斑：黄斑水肿为湿热蕴蒸、或脾肾阳虚、或阴虚火旺；黄斑区出血为脾虚不统血、或血热迫血妄行；黄斑区萎缩变性为气血两亏、或肝肾不足。

视网膜：视网膜出血量多且鲜红者，为血热迫血妄行，或肝阳上亢、或脾气虚弱；出血量少为阴虚火旺，或气血不足。

视网膜水肿为脾失健运、或肾阳不足，水湿上泛，或气郁血阻、或湿热蕴蒸。

视网膜渗出多由肺气不宣、或脾肾阳虚致痰湿内聚、或肝气郁结，气滞血淤所致。

视网膜退行性变多为耗气伤血、或肝肾不足。

玻璃体：玻璃体炎性混浊为浊气上犯、或阴虚火旺；出血性混浊为气滞血淤、或血热妄行、或外伤。

总之，眼底各组织的病理变化均为各脏腑功能失调的反应，因此眼底病的辨证，必须根据局部表现，结合全身症状进行全面分析，才能得出正确判断。

（蔡华松）

4 治疗概要

眼与脏腑、经络、气血关系密切。所以，自古以来医治内障眼病是以内治为主，强调从整体出发进行辨证，采用药物内服法。外障眼病则多配合外治，在眼局部直接施用药物及手术等治法。此外，还有针灸与按摩，亦为眼科所常用。

4.1 内治法

内治的各种方法，是在临床辨证求因的基础上，针对病因病机而设立的。眼科常用的内治法，自然也是针对眼科常见之病因病机而制定的。治法是立方遣药的依据，方药是治法的具体体现。眼科的内治法基本原则类似内科，但也有它某些特殊的内容。现将常用的内治法介绍如下。

疏风清热法

因风热所致的眼病，尤其是外障眼病最为多见。故疏风清热法是常用治疗原则之一。

风热之证除眼部出现红肿焮痛、羞明流泪，或痒，或眵多之外，间或伴有恶风、发热、头痛、脉浮数等全身性证候。治疗上给予疏风则表证解，清热则热证除。

泻火解毒法

本法是用性质寒凉的方药，通过泻火解毒，清除邪热的治法。主要用于热(火)证眼病。如胞肿如桃、疮疡疖肿、白睛混赤、黑睛溃陷、黄液上冲、瞳神紧小等。常伴有疼痛拒按、羞明流泪等眼症兼口渴、便秘、舌红、苔黄等全身症状。

眼科泻火解毒法为常用之治法。在具体应用时，由于病因病机不同，眼部所表现之火邪有肝火、心火、肺火、胃火、三焦火等之别，须根据脏腑辨证，灵活掌握。如眼胞焮肿赤痛，口渴喜饮，大便干燥，则用泻火通腑之法；抱轮红赤、黑睛生翳，眼球疼痛，苔黄脉弦之肝火上攻，则用清泻肝火法等。

本法容易损伤脾胃阳气，故不能久用，并要根据病情轻重和体质强弱，慎重选药。又因药性寒凉，久用可致气血凝滞，翳障难退，故对黑睛疾患，应用本法必须掌握尺度。属虚火者，则禁用此法。

滋阴降火法

本法是用滋养阴液，清降虚火的方法，解除阴虚火旺的证候，而达到明目效果的治法。主要适用于阴虚火旺的眼病。阴液亏损，虚火上炎，上攻于目，证见目微赤痛，眵泪稀薄，视物昏朦，兼见头目眩晕，失眠难寐，五心烦热，两颧潮红，盗汗梦遗，咳嗽痰血，烦躁善怒，口干舌燥，或耳鸣耳聋，或干呕、呃逆，或口舌生疮，或见低热，舌红而干，苔少，脉细数或虚数者。

虚火又有心、肺、胃、肝、肾等之分，临床上要结合脏腑辨证用药。如黑睛生翳，抱轮微赤，烦躁易怒，属肝经虚火；两眦血脉稀疏，心烦失眠，属心经虚火；白睛淡红，鼻干咽燥，属肺经虚火；瞳神干缺，眼底少量出血，耳鸣腰酸，五心烦热，属肾经虚火等。

补益肝肾法

本法是用具有补益肝肾作用的方药，以消除肝肾亏虚证候而达到明目作用的治法。虚证眼病多属肝肾不足。如外障的星点云翳，隐伏不显，白睛赤脉稀疏而色淡，冷泪常流；或内障的目无光彩，视物昏花，眼前蝇飞蚊舞，青盲，雀目等证，均可适用此法。

同时还须辨别其为肾阴虚损或肾阳亏虚。阴虚者着重补阴，阳虚者着重补阳，阴阳俱虚者，则阴阳双补。

益气补血法

本法是用具有补养气血作用的方药，以消除气血虚弱的证候，而达到明目作用的治法。眼病而属气血亏虚者，多外观如常，只有目光无神，视物昏矇或其他视觉上的变化，或仅有轻微干涩不舒，结膜微赤等证适用本法。

因气血相依，关系密切，故益气养血常同用。但亦应根据气血的偏重而灵活掌握。如兼见神疲、纳呆、胞睑下垂、开合乏力者，乃偏于气虚，应以益气为主。若因失血或久病，引起视物不明，头昏眼花，心悸失眠者，是偏于血虚，当以养血为主。由于脾胃为后天之本，气血生化之源，故补气养血时，常要兼顾脾胃。

邪气亢盛而无虚证者，忌用本法。

止血法

本法是运用具有止血作用的方药，以中止眼部出血的治法。适用于各种出血症的早期。如胞睑出血、白睛溢血、血灌瞳神、眼内出血等均可用本法。

根据不同的出血原因，止血的具体治法也有所不同。如血热妄行者，宜清热凉血止血；虚火伤络者，宜滋阴凉血止血；气不摄血者，宜益气摄血；眼外伤者，宜祛瘀止血等。

本法属急则治标之法，仅用于出血阶段，若出血已止，而无再出血的趋向，当逐渐用活血祛瘀法以促进瘀血的吸收，以免导致留瘀之弊。

活血化瘀法

本法是用具有活血祛瘀作用的方药，改善血行，消散瘀滞，促进眼部瘀血吸收的方法。凡眼睑青紫肿硬、白睛溢血、白睛紫胀肿起、眼内各个部位的瘀血、视网膜血管血流瘀滞或阻塞、眼部固定性疼痛及舌有瘀斑等，均属本法适应症。

气为血帅，气行则血行，故临床应用时，常配伍行气导滞药物，以提高疗效。孕妇忌用本法。

理气法

理气法包括补气和行气，前者在补益法介绍，本节仅限于行气法而言。本法是用具有调理气机作用的方药，以改善脏腑经络功能失调，气机运行受阻的病理情况，而达到明目作用的治法。

由于郁怒伤肝，疏泄失职，致肝气郁滞而生目疾者，颇为常见。其中尤以青风内障、绿风内障、视瞻昏渺等内障眼病为多。故无论内外障眼病，兼有胁胀、胸闷、嗳气、咽部似有物阻、急躁易怒、脉弦等症者，皆可用疏肝理气法治之。

肺气壅滞亦可致目疾。如白睛溢血或眼部浮肿而兼咳嗽不扬者，宜行气利肺法。

脾胃失调，气滞食积所致眼疾，当用行气消积导滞法，此外，若兼血淤眼证者，又当配伍活血祛淤之品。

气阴亏损者，慎用本法。

祛湿法

本法是用具有祛湿作用的方药，通过祛除湿邪，以治疗眼病的方法。凡水湿滞留脏腑经络而致的目疾，宜用本法。如眼睑水肿、睑弦湿烂、胞内粟疮、白睛污黄、翳如虫蚀、混睛障、云雾移睛、视瞻昏渺等，兼有头痛如裹、口不渴或口渴不欲饮、胸闷食少、腹胀便溏、四肢乏力，或咳吐痰涎等，为本法适应症。

因湿邪侵袭的部位和兼邪各有不同，故所用具体治法也有区别。如风湿犯眼，眼睑湿痒，则用祛风胜湿法；湿热上攻，眼睑红赤糜烂，湿痒交作，黑睛溃烂，则用清热祛湿法；痰湿阻滞，睑生肿核，或视物昏矇，眼前黑影飘动，眼底检查视网膜水肿、网膜、脉络膜有团状、点状渗出，兼见舌苔白腻、脉缓，则用化湿祛痰法；湿浊上泛，视网膜水肿，则用利水渗湿法；中焦虚寒，湿邪困滞见视物昏矇，或视瞻有色，兼见头目昏沉、身重怠倦、四肢不温，舌淡苔滑，脉沉迟，则用温中散寒，通阳利水法等。

退翳明目法

本法是用具有退翳作用的方药，以消退黑睛翳障，而达到明目作用的眼科独特治法。黑睛发生病变而现星点云翳者，适用本法。

退翳之法，须有层次，如病初起，星翳点点，红赤流泪，风热正盛，当以疏风清热为主，酌加退翳药。若风热渐减，则应在上述基础上，酌加退翳药。病至后期，风热已退，遗留翳障而正气已虚者，须在以退翳为主的基础上酌加益气养血或滋养肝肾等扶正之品。

黑睛属肝，故清肝、平肝、舒肝药物，亦有退翳作用，可配伍应用。黑睛生翳后期，以退翳为主，用药不可过于寒凉，以免攻伐太过，损伤正气，邪气冰伏，气血凝滞，翳不易退。

4.2 外治法

外治法为历代中医眼科主要治疗方法之一。凡直接用于眼或眼邻近部位以达治疗眼疾的方法，统属外治法。外治法临床应用甚为广泛。常与内治法密切配合，尤其是外障眼病，更是如此。内障眼疾，不少病类也强调配合外治法，如绿风内障、瞳神紧小、圆翳内障等，外治法是不可缺少的治疗环节。

外治法种类很多，除用药物点滴、熏洗、敷、熨外，也重视钩、割、烙、针等手术方法。现代中医眼科不仅继承了传统的外治法，而且积极改进，有所发展。现将几种常用的外治法简述如下：

1. 点眼法

本法是将药物直接点入眼部，是中医眼科常用外治法之一。凡胞睑溃烂、白睛红赤，肿痒、赤膜、白膜，黑睛生翳溃烂，瞳神紧小或干缺，五风内障，圆翳内障未成熟等，都可点药治之。常用的有眼药水，眼药膏与眼药粉三种。

2. 熏洗法

熏洗法是中医传统外治法之一。是利用药液煮沸后的热气蒸腾上熏眼部，熏后再用煎剂滤清液淋洗患眼。一般多先熏后洗，亦可只熏不洗。此疗法除具有湿热敷作用外，尚可通过不同药物直接作用于眼部，达到疏通经络，祛风清热，解毒消肿的效果。主要用于眼睑红肿，羞明涩痛、眵泪较多等外障眼。

3. 敷法

(1) 热敷：热敷能疏通经络、流通气血、有散瘀、消肿、止痛之功效。适用于外障眼病伴有目赤肿痛者，外伤24小时后的眼睑淤肿，白睛溢血和非新鲜性的血灌瞳神症等。脓成已局限病灶和有新鲜出血性眼疾，忌用本法。

(2) 冷敷：冷敷法有清热止痛，凉血止血作用。适用于眼睑外伤早期的皮下出血，或眼部的焮热肿痛。一般是用冰块或冷水毛巾外敷眼部。

(3) 药物敷法：药物敷法多选用有凉血止血、清热解毒、散瘀消肿止痛、祛风止痒等功效的不同药物，外敷于眼睑皮肤表面，适用于各种外障眼疾与外伤等。

4. 冲洗法

一般指结膜囊冲洗和泪道冲洗。适用于眵泪较多的白睛疾病，眼内化学液溅入，或结膜囊内异物及手术前清洁结膜囊等。后者用于探测泪道是否通畅及清除泪囊中积存的分泌物，或作为眼内手术前的常规准备。

5. 钩割法

本法是古代中医眼科常用手术方法。本法适用于翼状胬肉，眼部赘生物病症。手术时，首先用锋利之针穿入肉中，将胬肉挽起，方用锄刀逐步向黑睛和白睛分离，动作要轻，分离要干净，然后用刀割除，割毕以火烙，预防复发。其主要操作方法与近代胬肉切除术大体相似。

6. 烙法

本法是以特制之烙器在火上烧红，灼烙于眼病患处的治法。常用于钩割后，有预防病变复发及手术中止血作用。亦可用于睑弦赤烂，日久难愈者。熨烙时应注意保护好眼睑，眦部，黑睛等健康组织，熨烙温度不宜过高，以免灼伤深部组织。

7. 针法

常用的有三棱针法、铍针法、金针拨内障法。

(1) 三棱针法：此法是用三棱针刺穴位出血，或用于镰法，刺刮患部淤滞颗粒。作用开郁祛邪，逐淤消滞。适用于赤热肿痛之实证外障眼病。

(2) 铍针法：铍针两面有刃，尖如剑峰，可刺亦可切割。用于割除眼部胬肉及其他眼部赘生物；穿刺、切开已成脓之疮疡；剔除嵌于白睛、黑睛上之异物。

(3) 金针拨内障法：此法为中医眼科治疗圆翳内障的重要手术方法。用于年老体弱的圆翳内障患者，翳定障老时。现代医学在它的基础上，吸收西医同类手术的优点，建立了中西医结合的白内障针拨套出术。

方法：以左眼为例。术者坐于术眼同侧的前面，助手站在患者的左后方。先用缝线牵引下睑，助手用拉钩轻提上睑。

切口：用固定镊子夹持角膜缘 6 点处结膜组织，牵引眼球转向鼻上侧。在角膜缘外 4 毫米 4—5 点处，用三角形刀片垂直刺穿眼球壁，做一长约 3 毫米与角膜缘平行的切口。

拨障：断晶体悬韧带顺序如下：①先断 4—5 点处韧带：持拨障针使凹面向下，垂直插入切口约 3 毫米后，针头朝向 12 点，于睫状体与晶状体间轻摆前进，达瞳孔缘 12 点处，将针头凹面贴住晶状体，向下绕过赤道部拨断 4—6 点处悬韧带；②断颞上方韧带：将拨障针转到晶状体后下方放平针头，在相当于瞳孔区 1/3 处，自鼻侧向颞侧作水平摆动，划破玻璃体前界膜，然后转针凹面向下，退出 1/2 许，重新进针到晶状体前 1—4 点近赤道部，压晶状体向后下侧倾倒；③断鼻上方悬韧带，将针头进入到晶状体前 9—10 点处，压其向后下倾倒，以断 9—12 点悬韧带。晶状体成水平位时，拨障针再一次划破玻璃体前界膜；④断鼻下方悬韧带完成拨障，将拨针凹面抱住晶体鼻上方 9—10 点处赤道部，使12点处向颞下转移到眼球内颞下方之睫状体平坦部和视网膜锯齿缘附近，保留6点左右之悬韧带不断。

出针：起针后晶体不再浮起时即可出针。整复球结膜切口，使其覆盖巩膜切口。结膜下可适量注入激素及抗生素，扩瞳，单眼包扎。

注意点：拨针进入切口如有阻力感，要考虑到切口过小，或睫状体平坦部未被切透，或切口处有结膜组织带入。断颞下方韧带，拨针在越过晶状体下方赤道部时，针头切勿超过6点过多，以保持6点左右韧带不断，否则术毕，晶状体成游离状态，将随体位改变而移动，会影响上方视野。在划破玻璃体前界膜时，密切注意拨针不能伸入眼内过深，以免碰伤睫状体或视网膜锯齿缘。

4.3 眼科常用药物

内服药

1. 祛风药

风为百病之长，善行而数变，常易挟热、寒、湿、痰、入经入络，入腑入脏，为患多端，眼位至高，极易受风邪侵袭，故祛风药在眼科应用较广。由于祛风药性多辛散，易伤阴劫液，故凡阳盛火升，内热壅盛，阴虚血少，表虚多汗者，宜慎用。伤于内风者，也切不可妄投祛风药。

祛风药有祛风、消肿、止痛、止痒的作用。多用于外障眼病初期，出现目赤肿痛、刺痒、流泪、星翳初起等证。常用的有辛凉解表与辛温解表药两类。

(1) 辛凉解表药：常用的有桑叶、菊花、柴胡、薄荷、蔓荆子、葛根、蝉蜕等。桑叶菊花有疏散风热、清肝明目作用，二者常配伍应用于肝经风热眼病；柴胡有解热、舒肝、退翳、升提多种作用，通过不同配伍，可广泛应用于风热或肝热所致的黑睛翳障、绿风内障、瞳神紧小及由中气不足所致的上睑下垂、青盲内障等多种内外障眼疾；葛根解阳明之表，常用于风热眼疾兼有前额头痛者；蝉蜕疏散风热，明目退翳，止目痒，常用于黑睛翳障，及睑弦赤烂、椒疮、粟疮等有目痒症者。

其代表方为银翘散。

(2) 辛温解表药：常用的有荆芥、防风、羌活、白芷、独活、细辛、藁本等。荆芥、防风、羌活祛风止痛、止痒、消翳力量较强，三药常配伍应用于外感风寒所引起的目赤生翳，眼痛头痛，目痒难忍，三者不同之处是羌活偏祛风湿，风寒、风湿眼疾引起的眼疾、头痛皆可用之；荆芥有较轻度解热作用，且能理血疗疮；防风有通经活络、散结祛淤作用，常配活血药用于气血淤滞所致粟疮、火疳和外伤及手术后由淤血滞留所引起的疼痛；藁本治目痛而兼太阳巅顶头痛者。

其代表方为驱风一字散。

2. 清热药

目居清阳之位，为肝之窍，邪热易乘，肝火易犯，火性炎上，故眼病热证甚为常见。清热药性具寒凉，故适用于热毒火邪上攻于目所致的各种热性眼病。根据药性的不同，又可分清热泻火、清热解毒、泄热攻下、清热明目等药。

本类药性寒凉，易伤阳气，故凡眼病而见阳气不足，脾胃虚寒，大便溏泄者应慎用。苦寒药，久服易伤阴化燥，故眼病属阴虚者也应审慎。

(1) 清热泻火药：用于实热壅盛之火热目疾。常用的有石膏、知母、山栀子、桑白皮、黄连、黄芩、黄柏、淡竹叶、龙胆草等。其中黄连、淡竹叶泻心火，除心烦，适用于眦帷红赤；黄芩、桑白皮泻肺火，多用于白睛红赤；石膏、知母泻胃火，用于胞睑红肿与黄液上冲；山栀子泻三焦之火，配伍其他清热药，可广泛用于各种实热眼病；龙胆草泻肝胆实火，故常用于因肝火上炎所致的黑睛疾患；黄柏合知母可泻肾火，可用于退虚火，与黄连、黄芩配伍治湿热眼疾。

其代表方为泻心汤(泻心火)、泻肺汤(泻肺火)、通脾泻胃汤(泻胃火)、龙胆泻肝汤(泻肝火)。

(2)清热解毒药：用于一切火热毒邪所致实热目疾。常用的有金银花、连翘、野菊花、大青叶、板蓝根、蒲公英、紫花地丁等。因火毒所致眼疾各不相同，常根据症情辅用其他治疗法。如：有表邪者可酌加升麻、防风、荆芥之类疏风散邪药；眼红肿焮痛者，酌加丹皮、赤芍、大黄、乳香、没药等清热凉血活血止痛药；眼部疮痈成脓而不易溃穿者，酌加穿山甲、皂角刺等托毒透脓。

代表方为清热解毒汤。

(3) 通腑泻热药：用于阳明腑实，里热上攻引起的目赤肿痛、眵泪胶粘而兼大便秘结者。常用的有大黄、芒硝等。

其代表方为大承气汤。

(4) 清热凉血药：用于热邪入血入营所致之眼疾。常用的有犀角、元参、生地黄、丹皮、赤芍、紫草等。其中犀角、紫草凉血解毒、用于热毒炽盛所致血热妄行，视力骤降者；丹皮、赤芍清热凉血活血行淤，治血分郁热之目疾；生地黄、元参清热凉血，养阴生津，有血热妄行，阴虚液少者用之。

其代表方为清营汤。

(5) 清热明目药：主要用于风热所致之星点翳障。常用的有夏枯草、决明子、青葙子、密蒙花、木贼草等。夏枯草泻肝胆郁火，用于肝火所致目赤肿痛、眼底出血；决明子、青葙子清肝明目；密蒙花祛风热退目赤，养肝润燥；木贼草疏风清热，退翳明目。

其代表方为石决明散。

3. 补益药

眼病之虚证，多为气血虚或肝肾不足。故补益药中以益气养血及补益肝肾药较为常用。

(1) 益气养血药：益气药用于气虚所致之胞睑无力，常欲闭垂、凹陷不愈或青盲内障等。常用的有黄芪、人参、白术、山药、甘草等药。养血药用于血虚所致之眼干涩昏花、夜盲、青盲等症。常用的有熟地黄、当归、白芍、何首乌、阿胶、桑椹子等药。

益气药代表方为补中益气汤,养血药为四物汤。

(2) 补益肝肾药:用于肝肾不足所致之内外障眼病。本类药分为滋养肝肾和温补肾阳二类。滋养肝肾常用者如熟地、枸杞子、女贞子、复盆子、沙苑蒺藜、菟丝子、楮实子等。其中熟地黄滋阴力较强,为阴虚之内障眼疾首选药;枸杞子有滋补肝肾,益精明目作用,故广泛用于肝肾不足之内外障眼疾,常与菊花配伍应用;女贞子滋养肾阴、善治阴虚内热,常与具有滋补肾阴,凉血止血作用的旱莲草配伍用于眼内出血的早期;复盆子补肝肾,固精明目;沙苑蒺藜、菟丝子皆能补肾益精明目;楮实子平补肝肾,养肝明目。温补肾阳常用紫河车、鹿茸、巴戟天、淫羊藿、补骨脂、肉桂、附子等药。

代表方为六味地黄丸或右归丸。

4. 理血药

理血法主要是治理血分病变,眼科常见的血分病变有血溢、血淤、血热、血虚,宜分别用止血、活血化淤、凉血、补血法。后两法在清热药、补益药中已叙述。

(1) 止血药:适用于眼部各种出血症的出血阶段。根据出血原因和性质可分为凉血止血、收敛止血、温经止血和祛淤止血。

凉血止血用于血热妄行引起的眼内出血症之出血期。常用的有大蓟、小蓟、地榆、白茅根、旱莲草等。收敛止血用于各种眼病、眼外伤之新鲜出血未成淤者。常用的有仙鹤草、白芨、藕节、血余炭、百草霜等药。温经止血用于寒性出血者。常用的有艾叶、灶心土、荆芥炭等药。祛淤止血用于因淤血阻滞而出血者,本类药兼具止血及祛淤作用。常用的有三七、蒲黄、血竭、花蕊石、茜草等药。

其代表方为十灰散。

(2)活血化淤药：适用于眼部各种出血停止后，仍有淤血者，或淤血蓄滞所致的眼疾。常用的有桃仁、红花、泽兰、川芎、丹参、刘寄奴、王不留行、牛膝、赤芍、丹皮、乳香、没药、五灵脂、苏木、水蛭、䗪虫等。

其代表方为血府逐淤汤。

5. 理气药

理气法是以调理气机，使之恢复正常为主要作用的治疗方法。凡气机失调所致眼病，均可用理气药治疗。但理气药多辛温发散，易耗气伤阴，故兼阴虚者慎用。

理气药中眼科常用的为疏肝理气药、行气利肺药、行气导滞药三种。

(1) 疏肝理气药：用于情志不舒、肝气郁结所致之眼疾。如绿风内障、青风内障、视瞻昏渺、云雾移睛、青盲、暴盲等内障眼病。常用的有柴胡、青皮、香附、郁金、川芎、川楝子等药。

其代表方为逍遥散。

(2) 行气利肺药：用于肺失宣降，气机阻滞所致之白睛红赤，或肿胀高起，或白睛溢血等症。常用的有桑白皮、桔梗、前胡、旋复花、苏子、杏仁等药。常与地骨皮、枇杷叶等利肺药同用。

其代表方为泻白散。

(3) 行气导滞药：用于脾胃失调，内有积滞所致之胞睑红肿，痒痛生疮，或小儿疳积上目，或视瞻昏渺等症。常用的有枳实、陈皮、厚朴、木香、砂仁、沉香、莱菔子、槟榔等药。常与山楂、神曲、鸡内金等消食药同用。

其代表方为保和丸。

6. 祛湿药

祛湿药是运用芳香化湿、利湿、渗湿、苦寒燥湿、温阳利水等药物治疗因湿邪为患所致眼病的治法。芳香化湿、利水渗湿两类药为眼科常用药。

(1) 芳香化湿药：用于湿浊内阻所致的眼疾。常用的有藿香、佩兰、苍术、砂仁、白豆蔻、石菖蒲等药。

其代表方为藿香正气散。

(2) 利水渗湿药：用于水湿停蓄所致的眼疾。常用的有茯苓、猪苓、车前子、泽泻、滑石、薏苡仁、赤小豆等药。

其代表方为五苓散。

7. 化痰散结药

化痰散结药是用祛除或消除痰涎的药物，治疗由痰引起的眼疾，如胞生痰核，眼内痰聚而致的眼底水肿，渗出物较多，及眼瘤、鹘眼凝睛等症。常用的有温化寒痰和清热化痰两类。前者常用半夏、南星、白芥子、皂荚、旋复花等药。后者常用瓜蒌、贝母、葶苈子、礞石、海浮石、昆布、海藻等药。

其代表方为二陈汤、清痰饮。

8. 退翳明目药

本类药主要适用于邪气初退或邪气消退不久之黑睛云翳。一般疏散风热或清肝平肝的药物均有退翳作用。常用的有蝉蜕、秦皮、谷精草、木贼草、密蒙花、石决明、珍珠母、白蒺藜、青葙子、蛇蜕等药。其中蝉蜕、秦皮、谷精草、密蒙花退风热翳障；石决明、珍珠母、白蒺藜、青葙子退肝热翳障。退翳药大多性较和平，通过各种配伍可广泛用于各种新老翳障。

其代表方为石决明散。

常用的外用药：

1. 矿物类药：雄黄、朱砂、炉甘石、硼砂、玛瑙、石蟹、石燕等。

2. 动物类药：熊胆、猪胆、羊胆、鲭胆、麝香、牛黄、乌贼骨、蝉蜕、蛇蜕、石决明、珍珠母等。

3. 植物类药：银花、蒲公英、黄连、黄芩、黄柏、青黛、龙胆草、紫草、生地黄、菊花、薄荷、木贼、荆芥、防风、蒺藜、三七、乳香、没药等。

以上 3 类药可据其不同药性，制成眼科外用药剂，如水剂、膏剂、散剂、锭剂、膜剂等。

5 眼睑疾病

眼睑中医叫胞睑、眼脾。在五轮中属肉轮，在脏属脾，脾与胃相表里，所以眼睑疾病与脾胃有极密切的关系。如饮食不节，频食辛辣炙煿之品，则致脾胃失职，湿热内蕴，进而化火，上攻于目则眼睑为病。若中气下陷，气血亏虚，眼睑失养亦可致病。眼睑是眼睛的最外部分，易受外风毒邪侵袭，故其病来势急骤，局部症状明显。因此，在辨证时应局部与整体结合，辨明外邪内伤。属风热外袭者，治以疏风清热解毒为主；属脾胃火热上攻者，以清热泻火解毒为主；属湿热内蕴者，以清热利湿为主；内外合邪所致者，应内外兼治。

5.1 麦粒肿

麦粒肿是眼睑腺体(皮脂腺、睑板腺)的急性化脓性炎症，主要由葡萄球菌感染所致。因为发病部位不同，分内麦粒肿和外麦粒肿两种。麦粒肿中医称针眼，亦有土疳、土疡之称。

病因病机

多因风热时邪客于眼睑，血为邪乘凝而不行，血凝气滞于眼睑则发病；或因过食辛辣炙煿刺激性食物，致使脾胃蕴积热毒上攻于目而发病。

临床表现

初起眼睑疼痛，继则局部红肿，可触及硬节且压痛。外麦粒肿则在睫毛根部形成黄色或淡黄色脓头，内麦粒肿则在睑结膜面露出黄色脓头，若在外眦部常有球结膜充血、水肿。较重者有耳前淋巴结肿大与触痛。

辨证论治

1. 内治法

(1) 风热外束

主证：患眼异物感，恶风微痛羞明。眼睑轻微红肿，有硬节且压痛。微热恶风头痛，脉浮数，舌质淡红，苔薄白。

治法：疏风清热，佐以凉血。

方药：银翘散(1)加减。

金银花30克，连翘15克，薄荷9克，荆芥9克，桔梗9克，牛蒡子9克，野菊花12克，白芷6克，赤芍9克，炒黄芩9克，生甘草7克。水煎服，日1剂。

(2) 热毒内盛

主证：眼睑红肿疼痛较甚。肿块大或已成脓。耳前、颌下可触及肿大淋巴结且压痛。头痛，发热恶寒，口渴欲饮，便干、尿赤、脉洪数，舌质红苔黄。

治法：清热解毒，凉血散结。

方药：内疏黄连汤(2)加减。

黄连9克，黄芩9克，栀子9克，连翘15克，大黄6克，木香6克，薄荷9克，桔梗9克，赤芍9克，玄参6克，天花粉9克，白芷6克，制乳香6克，生甘草12克。水煎服，日1剂。

2. 其他疗法

(1) 用如意金黄散(84)调凡士林，涂患处，每日2次。

(2) 鲜生地黄适量，洗净捣烂取汁，与米醋同量和匀，涂患处，每日4次。

(3) 食盐、明矾适量，开水冲泡，澄清洗眼。

(4) 针刺放血疗法：取同侧耳背静脉，常规消毒，用三棱针浅刺之，每次1条静脉，出血为度，放血8~10滴。取少泽穴，用三棱针点刺出血。

(5) 针刺疗法：取穴合谷、攒竹、瞳子髎、鱼腰、四白。每日1次，每次取2穴，留针10分钟。

(6) 手术：脓成者，则切开排脓，勿挤压。
(7) 中成药：羚翘解毒丸(101)。每日服3次，每次9克。黄连上清丸(102)。每日服3次，每次6克。

5.2 眼睑脓肿

眼睑脓肿多由麦粒肿发展而来，也有因眶骨膜炎、眼睑丹毒、外伤引起者。中医称眼痈。

病因病机

胃火偏盛，又嗜食辛辣厚味之品，热郁化火，火热之邪上炎停留于眼睑肌肉组织之间且伤及营血，气血凝滞而酿脓发病；疮毒内陷，邪入营血，热毒蕴结，热壅血淤则肉腐，结聚为痈脓之变。

临床表现

眼睑红肿灼热剧痛。坚硬、触痛、球结膜充血、水肿或紫暗，耳前及颌下可触及肿大淋巴结。

辨证论治

1. 内治法

(1) 火热内盛

主证：眼症如上。头痛眼眶痛，发热恶寒，口渴欲饮，不思食物，唇干舌燥，大便干，尿黄赤，脉数有力，舌质红苔黄。

治法：清热泻火，解毒消肿。

方药：普济消毒饮(3)加减。

黄连9克，黄芩9克，金银花30克，连翘15克，板蓝根15克，玄参12克，牛蒡子12克，薄荷9克，桔梗9克，柴胡6克，当归12克，赤芍9克，苏木9克，生甘草9克。水煎服，日1剂。

(2) 疮毒内陷

主证：上述眼症。又眶周颜面漫肿，高热口渴，面红气短，脉洪大而数，舌质红绛或紫暗，舌苔黄稍厚。

治法：清营凉血，解毒消肿。

方药：清营汤(4)合五味消毒饮(5)加减。

生地黄 12 克，丹皮 9 克，黄连 6 克，连翘 12 克，金银花 30 克，野菊花 9 克，蒲公英 15 克，紫花地丁 12 克，淡竹叶 12 克，车前子 12 克，赤芍 9 克，制乳香 6 克，制没药 6 克，犀角粉 1.5 克。

犀角粉单煎或冲服。车前子用纱布包好，与其他药物一起水煎服，日 1 剂。

2. 其他疗法

(1) 川芎、当归、荆芥、皂刺、野菊花适量，水煎熏洗热敷、每日 3 次。

(2) 鲜芙蓉花叶洗净捣烂贴敷患处，每日 2 次。

(3) 中成药：牛黄解毒片(103)。每次 5 片，每日 3 次。

(4) 手术：脓已成者，切开排脓，勿挤压。

(5) 全身使用抗生素。

5.3 眼睑丹毒

眼睑丹毒是眼睑皮肤及皮下组织急性局限性炎症。由溶血性链球菌感染引起，多由面部蔓延而来，有传染性，起病急，并伴有发热、恶寒及毒血症。中医称眼丹。

病因病机

外感风热毒邪，侵袭眼睑，郁而不散则化热生火，热毒壅遏，气血结聚而发病；湿邪内蕴，郁而化热，脾经有风，风挟湿热而上行，滞于眼睑，湿热熏肤而发病。

临床表现

眼睑皮肤灼热，肿胀、充血。红肿区皮肤变厚隆起，呈现红色，表面有小水泡，病变区边界清晰，严重者局部坏死或向四周蔓延。常伴有发热、恶寒、头痛等全身症状。起病急剧。

辨证论治

1. 内治法

(1) 风热稽留

主证：眼睑红肿疼痛。局部皮肤高起增厚，色淡红，边界清晰。低烧，恶寒、头痛、鼻塞，全身不适，脉浮数，舌质淡红，苔薄白。

治法：祛风清热散邪。

方药：散热消毒饮子(6)加减。

黄连9克，黄芩9克，连翘15克，赤芍9克，川芎9克，郁金9克，牛蒡子12克，薄荷9克，白芷9克，防风9克，羌活9克，生甘草12克。水煎服，日1剂。

(2) 热壅湿盛

主证：眼睑疼痛剧烈，漫肿难开。皮厚灼热色紫暗，且有细小水泡。高热、恶寒或寒战，口渴不欲饮，小便赤涩，脉数，舌质红，苔黄腻。

治法：清热利湿，消肿止痛。

方药：黄连解毒汤(7)合三仁汤(8)加减。

黄连12克，黄芩9克，黄柏6克，栀子12克，滑石30克，淡竹叶12克，桔梗12克，薏苡仁15克，蔻仁9克，半夏9克，厚朴9克，川芎9克，细辛6克，羌活9克。 水煎服，日1剂。

2. 其他疗法

(1) 野菊花、薄荷、荆芥、赤芍水煎熏洗，每日2次。

(2) 芒硝、炉甘石适量，热开水冲泡，行湿热敷，每日4次。

(3) 青黛、香油适量，调成油糊状，涂患处。

(4) 耳针：取穴眼、肾上腺、内分泌、脾。每日针1次，每次留针10～15分钟。

5.4 眼睑湿疹

眼睑湿疹是一种以红斑、丘疹、水泡、渗出、鳞屑形成和结痂为特征的眼睑皮肤疾患。如果继发细菌感染，则局部可化脓而呈脓疱样改变。大多数由于对某种致敏物质或药物过敏引起。中医称风赤疮痍。

病因病机

湿毒邪气侵袭皮肤，郁遏卫表，清阳之气不能外达，皮肤失荣，且体内湿浊之气不降亦不得外泄，积聚久则发病；素体湿热内盛，湿热郁结不散则化火生风，风火相助挟湿上行，停于眼睑皮肌之间则发病。

临床表现

眼睑刺痒，烧灼感。眼睑皮肤红肿、有丘疹、小泡，继则渗出、糜烂、结痂。并可侵及球结膜、角膜，见球结膜充血、水肿、角膜表层浸润等。

辨证论治

1. 内治法

(1) 湿毒侵淫

主证：眼睑痒甚，痛轻，肿胀。皮肤见丘疹，小水泡，有渗出及糜烂。神疲懒倦，口中粘腻，脉濡缓，舌质胖色淡，苔白稍厚。

治法：化湿解毒，祛邪止痒。

方药：除湿汤(9)加减。

滑石30克，车前子15克，木通6克，白茯苓15克，黄芩9克，黄连9克，连翘15克，生甘草12克，炒苍术12克，薏苡仁30克，佩兰12克。车前子纱布包。水煎服，日1剂。

加减：若痒甚，加当归12克，赤芍9克。湿烂甚，加地肤子9克，苦参9克，白藓皮12克。

(2) 湿热并重

主证：眼睑肿胀疼痛而痒轻，烧灼感。皮肤充血、糜烂、腥臭、胶粘结痂。头昏如裹，身沉懒惰，大便灼热感，小便涩赤而痛，脉滑数，舌质红苔黄腻。

治法：清热利湿，凉血解毒。

方药：加减四物汤(10)。

生地黄12克，赤芍9克，当归9克，川芎9克，连翘15克，苦参15克，荆芥穗9克，防风9克，薄荷9克，徐长卿15克，炒苍术12克，猪苓9克，金银花15克，白藓皮15克，生甘草12克。水煎服，日1剂。

2. 其他疗法

(1) 用敷烂弦眼方(85)之药末，撒布于溃烂处。

(2) 穴位注射：取穴，大椎、肺俞、曲池、三阴交、膈俞。药物，维生素C100毫克或维生素$B_1$100毫克。每次选1,2个，每日注射1次。

5.5 霰粒肿

霰粒肿又称睑板腺囊肿，是睑板腺的慢性炎性肉芽肿。大多由于慢性结膜炎、睑缘炎引起睑板腺管道或排出口阻塞，导致腺体分泌物排出不畅或潴留所致。中医称胞生痰核。

病因病机

病人平素脾胃虚弱，又饮食不节或恣食辛辣醇酒厚味，伤及脾胃，脾健运失职，水湿停滞聚而为痰，痰湿阻络，稽留于眼睑皮肤肌肉之间，结聚日久则发病；湿痰停于脉络则血淤气滞而成症瘕而病；若痰湿郁结不散，湿遇阳气则化热，再外感风热，痰湿热三邪结聚，致淤血不行而发病。

临床表现

眼睑沉重不适或异物感，病程进展缓慢，眼睑皮下可触及豆粒大小圆形肿块。质硬不红肿，闭眼时眼睑皮肤稍隆起，皮肤与硬结不粘连，相应睑结膜呈局限性紫红色。

辨证论治

1. 内治法

(1) 痰湿郁滞

主证：患眼有异物感，或沉坠不适。眼睑皮肤隆起，触及硬结不痛。倦怠乏力，食欲不振，口中粘腻，脉细濡，舌质胖色淡，苔白腻。

治法：除湿化痰，活血散结。

方药：化坚二陈丸(11)加减。

清半夏9克，陈皮9克，白茯苓12克，黄连9克，昆布12克，白僵蚕6克，浙贝母12克，白芷9克，郁金9克，穿山甲9克。 水煎服，日1剂。

(2) 痰湿热结

主证：患眼异物感。局部隆起，触及硬节微痛，相应睑结膜充血，呈紫红色，脉濡稍数，舌质红，苔腻。

治法：清热利湿，软坚散结。

方药：防风散结汤(12)加减。

防风9克，独活6克，红花9克，苏木12克，当归9克，蒲黄9克，滑石30克，蚕砂12克，金银花30克，土茯苓15克，连翘12克，生甘草12克，丝瓜络15克。 水煎服，日1剂。

2. 其他疗法

(1) 野菊花、皂刺、红花、苏木各等分，水煎作湿热敷，每日3次。

(2) 用紫金锭(86)水调匀涂患处皮肤，每日2次。

(3) 手术：硬结较大，久不吸收者，切开刮除。

5.6 睑缘炎

睑缘炎是睑缘表面、睫毛毛囊及其腺体组织内亚急性或慢性炎症。多由细菌感染所致，最常见的为葡萄球菌、摩－阿氏双杆菌。另外，结膜的炎症，化学性或物理性刺激亦可诱发本病。中医称睑弦赤烂。

病因病机

病人过食辛辣厚味，脾胃蕴积湿热，湿热之气熏蒸眼睑，久则郁结不散而发病；风热毒邪外袭肌表，客于眼睑，致使毛孔闭塞，卫气不舒，卫外失职，皮肤失荣而致病。

临床表现

睑缘涩痒，或畏光流泪。在睫毛根部有糠麸样皮屑附着，或睑边漫生小脓疱，泡疹破裂，结痂，痂下是溃烂面，睑缘充血，肥厚，睫毛脱落，由于毛囊被破坏，睫毛不复生。也有在两眦部充血糜烂、常有刺痒感者。

辨证论治

1. 内治法

(1) 湿热毒盛

主证：畏光流泪，刺痛不止，或有搔痒感。睑缘红赤糜烂，胶粘溃陷出血，溢水湿烂。口干而粘腻，口渴不欲饮，脉濡稍数，舌质红，苔腻微黄。

治法：清热燥湿，祛风止痒。

方药：燥湿汤(13)加减。

黄连9克，栀子9克，苍术9克，白术12克，炒山药15克，陈皮9克，半夏9克，枳壳12克，胡黄连6克，秦皮9克，防风9克，白藓皮12克，地肤子12克，甘草9克。水煎服，日1剂。

(2) 风热外袭

主证：睑缘微红，奇痒，羞明。睫毛根部见糠麸样皮屑附着，睑缘充血。头痛恶风，咽干而痛，脉浮数，舌质红，苔薄黄。

治法：散风止痒，清热凉血。

方药：柴胡散(14)加减。

柴胡15克，荆芥9克，防风12克，羌活9克，赤芍9克，生地黄9克，桔梗9克，升麻6克，白藓皮12克，金银花15克，蒲公英15克，薄荷9克，荷叶9克，甘草9克。水煎服，日1剂。

(3) 脾虚挟湿

主证：睑缘轻微痒痛。睑缘红赤，多有湿疹样水泡，糜烂胶粘，或溢水湿烂。食欲不振，倦怠乏力，舌质淡体胖，苔白稍厚，脉濡弱。

治法：健脾渗湿。

方药：黄芪汤(15)加减。

黄芪30克，茯苓15克，炒山药15克，炒白术12克，升麻6克，炒枳壳9克，陈皮6克，防风9克，羌活9克，乌稍蛇6克，藿香12克，浮萍9克，甘草12克。水煎服，日1剂。

2. 其他疗法

(1) 千里光、野菊花、蒲公英、荆芥、防风、陈茶叶，水煎熏洗。每日3次。

(2) 野菊花、白矾，煎水澄清洗眼。每日3次。

(3) 凤凰油：鸡蛋1个，煮熟去白留黄，放勺内慢火煎熬成油，且频频搅动。用玻璃棒蘸少许涂患处。

(4) 蚕砂焙焦研细末，用香油或醋调成膏涂患处。

5.7 上睑下垂

上睑下垂是指上睑抬举困难，掩盖部分或全部瞳孔，影响视力的眼睑病。本病分先天性和后天性两种，本章重点讨论后天性睑下垂。其原因多由于提上睑肌或动眼神经受损害引起，及原因不明的重症肌无力。中医称上胞下垂，又称睑废。

病因病机

脾气亏虚，则输布失职，中气下陷，故精微物质不能输布于眼睑，睑失荣养则无力抬举；劳累汗出肌腠疏开，风邪乘机客于眼睑，邪留脉络则气血瘀阻不畅，使眼睑肌肤失养而致病。

临床表现

上睑下垂，抬举困难，有发于单侧者，亦有发于双侧者，轻者半掩瞳孔，重者上睑无力抬举，遮盖整个角膜，常有仰头视物的姿态。

辨证论治

1. 内治法

(1) 脾气亏虚

主证：常为双眼睑下垂，早晨轻，以后渐渐加重，休息轻或劳累后加重，有的可伴眼球运动障碍。精神疲乏，全身无力，舌质淡体胖有齿印，苔薄白，脉细弱。

治法：健脾升阳，补中益气。

方药：补中益气汤(16)加减。

黄芪30克，党参15克，炙甘草12克，白术15克，陈皮9克，升麻6克，葛根9克，柴胡12克，当归15克，白芍30克。 水煎服，日1剂。

加减：血虚者加鸡血藤30克，何首乌15克。下垂严重者，加川芎6克，丝瓜络15克，丹参30克，人参1.5克。大便稀者，加炮姜6克，熟附子6克。困倦，口中粘腻者，加佩兰15克，炒苍术12克，砂仁9克。

(2) 风邪入络

主证：起病突然。上睑下垂明显，多单眼发病，眼睑皮肤感觉减退或麻木不仁，眼球运动障碍。头痛头胀，舌质淡红，苔薄白，脉浮濇。

治法：祛风和血通络。

方药：助阳活血汤(17)加减。

黄芪30克，升麻9克，炙甘草9克，当归12克，白芍30克，柴胡15克，防风12克，葛根15克，钩藤12克，白芷9克，羌活9克。 水煎服。待水、药煮沸5分钟后，再放入钩藤。日1剂。

加减：舌质有瘀斑者，加丹参30克，郁金12克，鸡血藤30克，川芎6克。发热恶寒者，加金银花30克，连翘15克，薄荷9克。

2. 其他疗法

(1) 生姜切片烘热，熨贴眼睑皮肤。每日3次。

(2) 针刺：取穴，攒竹、丝竹空、鱼腰、足三里、脾俞、合谷。每次取眼周及远端穴各2个，每日针1次。

(3) 灸法：灸三阴交穴，每日1次，每次20分钟。

(4) 中成药：人参健脾丸(104)。

每日服3次，每次服9克。

(伊成运)

6 泪器疾病

泪器疾病属于中医两眦疾病的范畴。两眦在脏属心,属五轮中之血轮,所以两眦疾病多与心有密切关系。心主火,主血脉,心气盛则火炎,火炎则气血上壅逆行,使脉络郁阻,郁于眦部则发病。两眦暴露于外,易受风热火毒侵袭,搏结于此则发病。泪为肝液,所以以冷泪常流多与肝血不足,肝肾亏虚有关。在治疗两眦病时,多用清热散邪、清泻心火、温补肝肾之法。

6.1 泪道功能不全

泪道功能不全是指患者有泪溢而泪道无器质性病变,冲洗泪道通畅,但在结膜囊内滴入有色液体时,鼻腔中并无有色液体流出。流泪是由于泪液引流不畅或滞留所致。中医称冷泪症。

病因病机

多由肝肾两虚所致。五脏六腑皆有津液,通于目者为泪,肝所化液为泪,因此肝脏与泪液有密切关系。肝肾同源,肝肾虚弱,不能控制其液,则泪液外溢而致本病;血虚生风或外风侵袭,风性善动速变,血虚邪扰则泪器功能失常而发病。

临床表现

流泪不止,遇风更甚,但不畏光。眼睑松弛,眼轮匝肌软弱无力,泪囊张力差,可见泪小点与眼球接触不紧或冲洗泪道畅通或稍有阻力。

辨证论治

1. 内治法

(1) 肝肾虚弱

主证:肝肾虚弱,且眼干涩,视物模糊不清。头晕目眩,腰膝酸软，脉沉细，舌质红无苔。

治法：温补肝肾，收涩止泪。

方药：肾气丸(18)加减。

熟地9克，山萸肉9克，女贞子15克，山药9克，茯苓12克，肉桂6克，附子6克，肉苁蓉12克，菟丝子15克，五味子9克，麦冬12克，白芍15克，甘草9克。水煎服，日1剂。

(2) 血虚风扰

主证：平时双眼干涩而痒，常流泪，遇风时流泪不止，泪液清稀。口干唇燥，面色无华，脉沉弱，舌尖红少苔。

治法：养血生津，祛风止泪。

方药：止泪补肝散(19)加减。

当归15克，白芍18克，熟地黄9克，川芎6克，白蒺藜9克，防风9克，甘草9克，白藓皮9克。水煎服，日1剂。

加减：倦怠乏力者，加黄芪15克，党参12克。冬季泪多，畏寒，肢冷者，加细辛6克，桂枝12克。

2. 其他疗法

(1) 鲫鱼胆汁，新鲜人乳各等分，共调匀，少许点眼，每日3次。

(2) 针刺：取穴睛明、球后、承泣、阳白、肝俞、肾俞、合谷。每次取4穴，每日1次，留针20分钟。刺睛明穴时，进针至鼻骨处，行雀啄法，至有酸麻胀感为度，留针20分钟。

(3) 中成药：杞菊地黄丸(110)。每日服3次，每次服9克。

十全大补丸(105)。每日服3次，每次服9克。

6.2 慢性泪囊炎

慢性泪囊炎以挤压泪囊部有粘液脓性分泌物从泪小点溢出为特征。由于鼻泪管阻塞，泪液长期滞留于泪囊内，造成泪囊粘膜充血、肥厚、细菌生长繁殖所致。中医称漏睛。

病因病机

暑湿之邪侵袭泪窍，或脾蕴湿热，循太阳膀胱经上行，滞留内眦，积久热腐化脓致病；气血亏虚，风热侵入泪窍，无力祛邪外出，日久化脓致病。

临床表现

泪溢不止，时有流脓。泪囊部皮肤色泽正常，挤压则见粘液性或脓性分泌物从泪小点外溢，有的泪囊部可触及波动性囊肿，泪道冲洗不通。

辨证论治

1. 内治法

(1) 湿热滞留

主证：自觉内眦部胀涩不适，时时流泪，泪液呈胶粘状。睑裂内积泪较多，挤压泪囊部有大量泪液或脓性分泌物外溢。头沉胸闷，口渴不欲饮，脉滑稍数，舌质红，苔腻微黄。

治法：清热利湿，活血排脓。

方药：泻脾除热饮(20)加减。

黄连9克，黄芩9克，大黄3克，芒硝6克，黄芪15克，白芷6克，制乳香9克，桔梗9克，淡竹叶12克，金银花30克，连翘15克，生甘草12克。 水煎服，日1剂。

(2) 正虚邪留

主证：流泪不止，泪液清稀或胶粘。泪囊部皮肤色泽正常，挤压泪囊部流出分泌物为清稀泪液或稀脓样，缠绵日久。倦怠乏力，大便稀，脉细弱，舌质淡，苔白薄。

治法：扶正排脓，清热祛邪。

方药：千金托里散(21)加减。

黄芪24克，党参12克，茯苓12克，葛根12克，白芍15克，当归9克，川芎9克，桔梗9克，皂刺6克，甘草9克。水煎服，日1剂。

2. 其他疗法

手术：治疗无效者，行鼻腔泪囊吻合术，或泪囊摘除术。

6.3 急性泪囊炎

急性泪囊炎是泪囊急性化脓性炎症。可在慢性泪囊炎的基础上继发感染引起,亦可以并无泪道阻塞而突然发病。中医叫漏睛疮。

病因病机

风热毒邪袭表后,循太阳之经上行而滞留于内眦;心经蕴热,日久热入血脉,上攻内眦,久则热壅肉腐而发病。

临床表现

内眦泪囊部疼痛剧烈,灼热感,疼痛可放射至额部。常伴有头痛、发热、恶寒,全身不适。泪囊部高度红肿,其周围皮肤也充血肿胀,泪囊部可触及硬块,明显压痛,颌下及耳前淋巴结肿大。

辨证论治

1. 内治法

(1) 风热壅盛

主证:流泪疼痛并作。泪囊部皮肤充血肿胀,压痛,可触及硬结。咽痛鼻干,恶风发热,脉浮数,舌质红,苔薄黄。

治法:疏风清热、泻火凉血。

方药:竹叶泻经汤(22)加减。

淡竹叶12克,黄连9克,大黄3克,栀子9克,黄芩9克,泽泻9克,茯苓12克,柴胡9克,白芷9克,防风9克,桔梗9克,金银花30克,连翘15克,蒲公英30克。水煎服,日1剂。

(2) 热毒炽盛

主证:泪囊部疼痛剧烈,灼热感。局部皮肤充血紫暗、肿胀,并向周围扩展,触及肿块而拒按,颌下或耳前可触及肿大淋巴结。发热恶寒,口干而渴,脉洪大有力,舌质红,苔黄。

治法:清热解毒,泻火消肿。

方药：内疏黄连汤(2)加减。

黄连9克，黄芩9克，栀子9克，连翘12克，薄荷9克，桔梗9克，大黄3克，白芷9克，制没药6克，苏木9克，野菊花12克，牛膝9克，玄参9克，生甘草9克。 水煎服，日1剂。

2. 其他疗法

(1) 未成脓者，可用紫金锭(86)外涂，每日2次。

(2) 鲜野菊花15克，红糖适量，共捣烂，外敷患处，每日2次。

(3) 金银花30克，野菊花15克，苏木9克，水煎湿热敷，每日3次。

(4) 手术：脓已成者，切开排脓，成瘘管者，待炎症控制后，摘除泪囊。

(5) 中成药：牛黄清心丸(106)。每次服9克，每日3次。

(伊成运)

7 结膜疾病

结膜居眼球之外表,易受外邪致病因素的影响而发病。球结膜属中医白睛范畴,睑结膜属中医眼睑范畴,白睛在脏属肺,为气轮,眼睑在脏属脾,为肉轮,所以结膜疾病与肺、脾有密切关系。多由肺气不宣,肺阴不足,脾经湿热所致。在治疗上,多用疏风清热,宣通肺气、养阴润肺,清利湿热之法。

7.1 沙眼

沙眼是由沙眼衣原体感染引起的慢性传染性结膜炎症。偶然可急性发作,然后进入慢性炎症过程,后期可发生许多并发症,甚而致盲。中医称椒疮。

病因病机

湿热内蕴,复感风热毒邪,湿热交阻,随风热之邪蒸腾于目,使眼睑脉络壅滞,气滞血瘀而发病;中焦热盛,移热脉络,血热壅盛,致眼睑脉络瘀阻而发病。

临床表现

沙眼轻者多无自觉症状,或有轻微异物感,迎风流泪,分泌物稍多。较重者或有合并症者可有畏光流泪,分泌物粘着,视疲劳。可见上睑结膜及穹窿部肿胀充血,血管不清晰,结膜表面高低不平,乳头肥大,滤泡增生。早期可见角膜上缘血管翳与灰白色浅层浸润,结膜肥厚,见粗细不等之灰白色网状疤痕。后期可产生上睑下垂、内翻倒睫、角膜溃疡、角膜血管翳、睑球粘连、眼球干燥及泪囊炎等。

辨证论治

1. 内治法

(1) 湿热内蕴

主证：眼痛干涩，异物感，羞明多泪，分泌物粘着。眼睑轻度肿胀，睑结膜乳头肥大成片，滤泡增生较多，球结膜轻度充血，角膜血管翳。精神不振，不思饮食，口中粘腻，脉滑数，舌质红，苔黄腻。

治法：清热除湿，凉血散瘀。

方药：除风清脾饮(23)加减。

荆芥穗9克，桔梗12克，防风9克，黄连9克，连翘15克，知母6克，玄明粉6克，大黄3克，陈皮9克，石膏30克，生地黄9克，秦皮9克，甘草12克。水煎服，日1剂。

加减：眼痒甚者，加白蒺藜12克，白藓皮9克，苦参9克。睑内红赤显著者，加丹皮9克，赤芍9克，苏木9克。

(2) 风热偏盛

主证：眼干涩，异物感，痒而微痛，迎风流泪。睑结膜见细小乳头，滤泡少许。口干咽痛，脉浮数，舌质红，苔薄黄。

治法：疏风清热，凉血止痒。

方药：清脾凉血汤(24)加减。

防风12克，荆芥9克，白藓皮9克，蝉蜕9克，白菊花9克，地肤子9克，陈皮9克，苍术9克，厚朴6克，连翘15克，赤芍9克，大黄3克，丹皮9克，甘草9克。水煎服，日1剂。

(3) 热毒内盛

主证：羞明、流泪。刺痛严重，分泌物多。睑结膜充血，弥漫性乳头肥大，滤泡增生，球结膜充血，角膜血管翳明显。大便干结，尿黄赤，口渴喜饮，脉数大，舌质红，苔黄。

治法：清热泻火，凉血祛瘀。

方药：归芍红花散(25)加减。

当归12克，赤芍9克，红花9克，大黄3克，生地黄9克，黄芩9克，栀子9克，连翘12克，板蓝根15克，徐长卿

15克，防风9克，白芷9克，甘草9克。 水煎服，日1剂。

2. 其他疗法

(1) 用外障眼药水(87)，点眼，每日4次。

(2) 黄连西瓜霜眼液(88)点眼，每日4次。

(3) 桑白皮、枯矾、青盐等量，水煎澄清洗眼。

(4) 针刺：取足三里、血海、太冲穴，每日针1次，强刺激。

7.2 急性卡他性结膜炎

急性卡他性结膜炎，以明显的结膜充血，有粘液脓性分泌物为特征。多由葡萄球菌、肺炎球菌、链球菌及科-韦氏杆菌引起，为直接接触传染。中医称暴风客热。

病因病机

风热毒邪侵袭肌表，温邪上袭，首先犯肺，肺经风热上炎于目而发病；病人素体内热阳盛，再外受风热之邪，内外合邪，上炎于目则发病。

临床表现

有异物感，重则灼热疼痛，畏光流泪，眼眵多，甚者晨起睑裂全被封闭。睑结膜充血，眼睑肿胀，球结膜充血或有水肿，结膜下可见点状、片状出血。

辨证论治

1. 内治法

(1) 风热偏重

主证：患眼痒涩异物感，羞明流泪不止，分泌物较少而稀。眼睑轻微红肿，球结膜充血。头痛、鼻塞、恶风、微热，脉浮数，舌质淡红，苔薄白。

治法：宣肺疏风，清热凉血。

方药：驱风散热饮子(26)加减。

牛蒡子12克，羌活9克，防风9克，薄荷9克，菊花9

克，冬桑叶9克，连翘12克，栀子9克，大黄3克，赤芍9克，当归9克，川芎6克。 水煎服，日1剂。

(2) 肺热偏盛

主证：畏光流泪，灼热疼痛，分泌物多而粘稠。眼睑浮肿，球结膜水肿，充血呈鲜红色。口渴，咽干咳嗽，大便干，脉数，舌质红，苔薄黄。

治法：清热泻火，疏风散邪。

方药：泻肺饮(27)加减。

石膏30克，黄芩12克，桑白皮9克，麦冬9克，栀子9克，连翘15克，茯苓9克，木通9克，羌活9克，浮萍12克，菊花9克，丹皮9克，赤芍12克，甘草9克。 水煎服，日1剂。

(3) 肝肺火盛

主证：眼症同前。另外角膜的浅层可见灰白色点状混浊。胁痛、口苦咽干，脉弦数，舌边红，苔薄黄。

治法：清肝泻火，宣肺凉血。

方药：清肝散(28)加减。

黄芩9克，龙胆草9克，柴胡9克，丹皮9克，桑白皮9克，地骨皮9克，生地黄9克，大黄6克，薄荷9克，荷叶9克，桔梗9克，葶苈子9克，当归9克，羌活6克。 水煎服，日1剂。

2. 其他疗法

(1) 桑叶9克，菊花9克，硼砂3克，胆矾3克。水煎熏洗，每日3次。

(2) 10—50%千里光眼药水(89)点眼。

(3) 针刺：取穴太阳、四白、曲池、合谷，每日针1次，强刺激。

(4) 点刺放血：取耳后静脉3条，角孙、太阳、耳尖穴。任选1处，常规消毒，用三棱针点刺，挤出血3滴，每日1次。

7.3 流行性急性结膜炎

流行性急性结膜炎以发病急,传染性强,球结膜水肿及出血为其特征。由肠道病毒或腺病毒引起。中医称天行赤眼。

病因病机

外感疫疠毒邪,沿肺经上犯于目,或疫疠毒邪直接侵袭于目所致;肺胃热盛,又疫疠之气外袭,内外合邪交攻于目而发病。

临床表现

畏光流泪,头痛,眼眶痛。眼睑红肿,球结膜充血水肿,球结膜下见点状、片状出血,分泌物较少而呈粘性,角膜浅层点状浸润,吸收缓慢,耳前淋巴结肿大。

辨证论治

1. 内治法

(1) 疫毒侵袭

主证:畏光流泪,异物感。球结膜充血水肿。头痛,眼眶痛,恶风,全身疲乏无力,脉浮,舌质红,苔薄白。

治法:疏风散疫,清热解毒。

方药:普济消毒饮(3)加减。

板蓝根30克,马勃9克,牛蒡子9克,薄荷9克,菊花9克,柴胡9克,桔梗9克,桑白皮9克,连翘15克,黄连6克,黄芩9克,土茯苓15克,甘草9克。 水煎服,日1剂。

(2) 热毒炽盛

主证:畏光流泪,热泪如汤。眼睑浮肿,球结膜高度充血水肿,球结膜下出血,耳前腺肿大压痛。口渴喜饮,大便干结,脉洪大,舌质红,苔黄燥。

治法:清热泻火,解毒散疫。

方药:清瘟败毒饮(29)加减。

石膏30克,知母9克,甘草9克,黄连9克,黄芩9克,栀子9克,连翘12克,赤芍9克,丹皮9克,生地黄12克,桔梗9克，蚤休15克，大青叶6克，薄荷9克。 水煎服，日1剂。

2. 其他疗法

(1) 1%黄芩素眼液(90)点眼。

(2) 板蓝根或大青叶15克，水煎过滤，熏洗眼。

(3) 针刺放血：取耳后静脉3条，常规消毒，用三棱针点刺，挤出血5滴，每日1次。

7.4 慢性卡他性结膜炎

慢性卡他性结膜炎以眼睛干涩而痒，睑结膜轻度充血为其特点，病程长而顽固。多由微生物感染和化学或物理因素刺激所致。中医称白涩症。

病因病机

肺阴不足，阴虚火动则肺清肃之令不行，再外感风热之邪，风热挟虚火上炎于目而致病；风热侵袭，余热未清，潜伏肺脾之络，遇机则上炎发病；脾胃湿热内蕴，清气不升，湿热熏蒸，目失荣养而发病。

临床表现

双眼痒，异物感，干燥烧灼感，喜欢闭目。两外眦角有白色泡沫样分泌物，睑结膜轻度充血，乳头肥大，甚则睑结膜呈绒状粗糙状态。

辨证论治

1. 内治法

(1) 肺阴不足外感风热

主证：眼干涩不适，痒而眵少，微畏光流泪。睑结膜轻度充血。咽干口燥，脉浮细，舌质红，苔白薄。

治法：养阴清肺，疏风清热。

方药：桑白皮汤(30)加减。

桑白皮12克，麦冬9克，玄参9克，地骨皮12克，黄芩9

克，旋复花9克，菊花9克，桔梗9克，荷叶9克，山豆根9克，天花粉12克，防风9克，甘草9克。

水煎服，旋复花用布包，日1剂。

(2) 湿热蕴积

主证：眼沙涩烧灼感，畏光流泪。睑结膜充血，乳头肥大，球结膜轻度充血。尿黄，脉濡数，舌质红，苔黄腻。

治法：清利湿热，宣畅气机。

方药：三仁汤(8)加减。

滑石30克，半夏9克，杏仁6克，薏苡仁15克，蔻仁9克，淡竹叶9克，桑白皮9克，泽泻9克，茯苓9克，赤芍9克。 水煎服，日1剂。

(3) 余邪隐伏

主证：眼干涩，轻微灼热感，午后或夜间甚，目痒眵少。睑结膜轻度充血。干咳咽痛，脉浮稍数，舌质红，苔薄黄。

治法：清肺经伏热。

方药：泻肺汤(31)加减。

桑白皮15克，麦冬12克，地骨皮9克，黄芩9克，知母9克，桔梗9克，薄荷9克，菊花9克，浙贝母9克，连翘9克，炒当归12克，甘草9克。 水煎服，日1剂。

2. 其他疗法

(1) 桑叶9克，白菊花9克，水煎熏洗眼。

(2) 犀黄散(91)点眼。

7.5 泡性结膜炎

泡性结膜炎是一种局限性的球结膜炎症，由结膜上皮组织对某种致敏毒素所表现的迟发性变态反应，多见于体质差的儿童。中医称金疳。

病因病机

燥邪犯肺，郁而化热，燥热郁结则肺之宣发失职，致血脉瘀滞而致病；素体肺阴不足，燥邪袭之更伤阴，虚火上炎，肺络壅阻，气滞血瘀而致病。

临床表现

异物感，微痛稍痒，微羞明流泪。球结膜上见灰白色泡疹，也可在角结膜缘，泡疹周围局限性充血。

辨证论治

1. 内治法

(1) 燥热郁结

主证：沙涩感，微痛，羞明流泪。球结膜上见一淡红白色泡疹，其周局限性充血。口渴干燥，脉稍数，舌质红干裂，苔薄黄。

治法：润肺散结，清热凉血。

方药：清燥救肺汤(32)加减。

石膏30克，知母9克，桑叶9克，杏仁3克，枇杷叶9克，麦冬12克，瓜蒌12克，火麻仁12克，丹皮9克，赤芍9克，炙百合9克，甘草9克。 水煎服，日1剂。

(2) 阴虚邪恋

主证：眼部症状同前，且反复发作，口干咽燥，干咳，脉细，舌质红苔少。

治法：养阴润燥，宣肺透邪。

方药：冶金汤(33)加减。

玄参12克，桑白皮9克，杏仁3克，黄连9克，黄芩9克，葶苈子12克，天花粉12克，菊花9克，防风9克，枳壳9克，桔梗12克，甘草9克。 水煎服，日1剂。

2. 其他疗法

(1) 红花9克，金银花30克，丝瓜络9克，水煎熏洗，每日3次。

(2) 耳针：取内分泌、眼、交感、神门穴，每日针1次，5分钟捻转1次，留针20分钟。

7.6 春季卡他性结膜炎

春季卡他性结膜炎是一种因过敏引起的有特殊形态的结膜间质增殖性炎症。分睑结膜型、球结膜型和混合型。其特点是每逢春夏季节病势加剧，秋冬可自行缓解，来年春季又发。过敏源多为物理性因素。中医称目痒或时复症。

病因病机

脾经湿热内蕴，又加外感风热时邪郁于肺，风热挟湿热上攻于目，搏结眼睑、结膜，致脉络瘀塞不通而发病；患者血虚，血虚则风邪乘虚而入。血虚亦生内风，内外合邪上攻于目则发病。

临床表现

眼部奇痒，烧灼感，异物感，畏光流泪。分泌物呈粘丝状，睑结膜充血明显，硬而扁平的乳头满布睑结膜，似鹅卵石路面样，亦可表现为球结膜充血，色素沉着，呈污秽的黄红色，角膜缘发生灰黄色胶样肥厚，或两者兼有。

辨证论治

1. 内治法

(1) 脾经湿热　风热外束

主证：眼部症状悉俱，嗜睡，口中粘腻，不思饮食，脉浮，舌质红，苔腻微黄。

治法：清热利湿，祛风止痒。

方药：消风除热汤(34)。

黄芩9克，栀子9克，秦皮9克，柴胡12克，前胡9克，防风9克，白芷9克，薄荷12克，大黄3克，苦参12克，葛根12克，石膏15克，徐长卿30克，甘草9克。　水煎服，日1剂。

(2) 血虚风袭

主证：眼部奇痒，干涩难忍，羞明流泪，遇风更甚。睑结膜充血，血管不清晰，球结膜轻度充血，色污秽。面色少华，倦怠乏力，脉沉细，舌质淡红少苔。

治法：养血祛风，活血止痒。

方药：当归活血饮(35)加减。

当归15克，熟地黄9克，白芍15克，川芎9克，羌活9克，薄荷9克，防风9克，赤芍9克，黄芪15克，苍术9克，甘草9克，茯苓12克，党参9克。水煎服，日1剂。

2. 其他疗法

(1) 春雪膏(92)点眼，每日3次。

(2) 针刺：取睛明、太阳、合谷、足三里穴，每日1次，中度刺激。

7.7 翼状胬肉

翼状胬肉是由于球结膜上皮组织变性、增厚而形成的、向角膜方向生长的三角形粘膜皱襞，多位于睑裂部，可分为进行性和静止性翼状胬肉。中医称胬肉攀睛。

病因病机

心火炽盛，火盛则生风，风火相助其势上炎于目内眦而发病，风热外袭，先犯于肺，肺经风热上攻目内眦亦可致病。

临床表现

眼干涩而痒。内眦部球结膜充血肥厚，呈三角形，其尖端向角膜进行，形成胬肉，可分头、颈、体三部分。头部尖而呈灰白色胶样隆起，颈体部肉样充血，组织肥厚，则为进行性的。若头部平坦，颈体部血管收缩，组织菲薄，则为静止性的。

辨证论治

1. 内治法

(1) 心火炽盛

主证：眼沙涩不适，胬肉充血肥厚，有眵而干结。心烦口渴，口舌生疮，小便少而赤，脉数，舌尖红苔黄。

治法：清心泻火，凉血散瘀。

方药：泻心汤(36)加减。

黄连9克，连翘15克，莲子心3克，淡竹叶12克，甘草12克，生地黄9克，赤芍9克，当归9克，茺蔚子12克，石膏30克，荆芥穗9克，防风9克，郁金9克。水煎服，日1剂。

(2) 肺经风热

主证：眼涩痒。胬肉色红，头尖而隆起，进行较快。咽干咳嗽，脉浮数，舌质红，苔薄黄。

治法：宣肺疏风，清热活络。

方药：泻肺饮(27)加减。

黄芩9克，桑白皮9克，地骨皮9克，栀子12克，连翘15克，木通6克，甘草9克，薄荷9克，菊花12克，防风9克，生地黄12克，玄参9克，丹皮9克。水煎服，日1剂。

(3) 阴虚火旺

主证：胬肉淡红，头部平坦。心中燥热，口干舌燥，脉沉细，舌质红少苔。

治法：滋阴降火。

方药：滋阴降火汤(37)加减。

生地黄12克，麦冬9克，知母9克，黄柏6克，黄芩9克，当归9克，熟地黄9克，白芍12克，甘草9克，柴胡9克，泽泻9克，沙参9克。水煎服，日1剂。

2. 其他疗法

必要时，手术切除。

(伊成运)

8 巩膜疾病

巩膜具有保护球内容物的功能，属中医白睛范畴，白睛在脏属肺为气轮，所以巩膜病与肺关系密切，治以清热润肺，宣肺祛邪为主。

8.1 巩膜炎

巩膜炎根据病变部位的深浅，可分为浅层巩膜炎，巩膜炎（即深层巩膜炎）两种，病情严重者，可引起角膜及葡萄膜的并发症，其病因主要是内源性因素，本质上均属胶原纤维病范畴，中医称火疳。

病因病机

肺热壅盛，宣降失职，气机不利，气滞血瘀，脉络阻塞，发于白睛而致病；心火内盛，肺为娇脏，肺受心火灼烁则白睛发病；湿热内蕴，兼受风邪，风挟湿热蒸腾于目，血脉瘀阻而发病。

临床表现

眼异物感，畏光流泪，眼球疼痛，夜间尤甚。局限性巩膜充血，呈紫红色或紫蓝色，见结节性或稍弥漫性隆起，压痛明显，炎症可累及角膜及虹膜。

辨证论治

1. 内治法

(1) 肺热壅盛

主证：眼羞明流泪疼痛。巩膜浅层充血呈紫红色，见结节隆起。口干咽痛咳嗽，脉数，舌质红，苔薄黄。

治法：清热宣肺，活血散结。

方药：桑白皮汤(30)加减。

桑白皮15克，麦冬9克，玄参9克，地骨皮12克，黄芩9克，菊花9克，桔梗9克，葶苈子9克，薄荷9克，牛蒡子12克，浙贝母9克，赤芍9克，红花9克，夏枯草15克。水煎服，日1剂。

(2) 心火亢盛

主证：羞明流泪，眼球胀痛。巩膜充血紫暗，局部弥漫性隆起。口舌生疮，小便短赤，脉稍数，舌质尖红，苔薄黄。

治法：清心泻火，凉血散结。

方药：泻心汤(36)加减。

黄连9克，连翘12克，生地黄12克，赤芍9克，淡竹叶9克，甘草9克，大黄3克，木通9克，制乳香9克，制没药9克，苏木9克，皂刺9克。水煎服，日1剂。

(3) 风湿热邪攻目

主证：羞明流泪疼痛。巩膜充血色暗红。头痛胸闷，关节疼痛，脉滑，舌质稍红，苔白厚。

治法：祛风胜湿，清热散结。

方药：散风除湿活血汤(38)加减。

羌活9克，独活9克，防风9克，前胡12克，白术9克，忍冬藤15克，当归9克，赤芍12克，鸡血藤30克，红花9克，赤茯苓9克，枳壳9克，桔梗9克，甘草9克。水煎服，日1剂。

2. 其他疗法

(1) 五胆膏(93)点眼。

(2) 穴位注射：取瞳子髎、睛明、四白、鱼腰穴，以0.5%普鲁卡因作穴位注射。每日1次，每穴0.25毫升。

(3) 中成药：养阴清肺丸(107)。

每日服3次，每次服9克。

(伊成运)

9 角膜疾病

角膜疾病的特点其一因本身无血管,营养供应较差,新陈代谢缓慢,病变修复慢,病程长;其二角膜质地透明,病变痊愈后,遗留瘢痕混浊,不同程度影响视功能。

角膜在五轮中属风轮,内应于肝,肝胆相表里,故角膜病辨证多从肝胆着手。本病早期多为肝经风热,或肝经实热;病变后期,或反复发作,或时轻时重多为肝阴不足。在治疗时除按辨证选方外,应酌情加退翳明目药,以促进视功能恢复。

9.1 匐行性角膜溃疡

本病是化脓性角膜溃疡,常由肺炎双球菌、葡萄球菌等感染所致。溃疡常向角膜中央匐行,并伴有前房积脓,故又称前房积脓性角膜溃疡。中医称凝脂翳。

病因病机

角膜表层外伤,风热毒邪乘机而入;肝胆火盛,上攻于目,致气血壅滞,蓄腐成脓而患病;也可由其他角膜炎复感邪毒演变而来。

临床表现

眼有异物感、疼痛、畏光流泪,视物模糊。检查见睫状充血或混合性充血,初起角膜出现灰白色浸润点,浸润扩大加深而成溃疡。由于虹膜受刺激,产生房水混浊及前房积脓,严重者,角膜溃疡向深部发展导致穿孔,多数病例形成粘连性角膜白斑而痊愈,少数较重者可形成角膜葡萄肿,或眼球内容炎,或全眼球炎而致失明,眼球萎缩。

辨证论治

1. 内治法

(1) 风热壅盛

主证：初起有轻微异物感，羞明流泪，视力减退，睫状充血，角膜中央浸润，兼头痛，舌红，苔薄白或薄黄，脉浮数。

治法：疏风清热。

方药：新制柴连汤(39)加减。柴胡9克，蔓荆子9克，荆芥9克，防风9克，黄芩9克，栀子9克，龙胆草9克，木通6克，木贼草12克，赤芍15克，甘草6克。水煎服，日1剂。

(2) 肝胆火炽

主证：眼痛、羞明流泪、视物模糊明显加重，混合性充血，角膜溃疡，前房积脓，伴口干咽燥，便秘尿赤，舌红苔黄，脉弦数。

治法：清肝泻火。

方药：龙胆泻肝汤(40)加减。龙胆草、栀子、黄芩、柴胡、泽泻、木通、车前子各9克，生地黄15克、当归12克，谷精草12克。用法：水煎服，日1剂。

加减：便秘加大黄9克，芒硝9克，心烦口渴加石膏15克，知母9克；眼痛重加赤芍15克，红花9克。

(3) 正虚邪留

主证：症状缓解，角膜溃疡面部分修复，或病程长，病情轻，但久不愈，舌质淡，脉弱。

治法：扶正祛邪。

方药：托里消毒散(41)加减。黄芪30克、川芎9克、当归、白术、茯苓、人参各12克、金银花18克、白芷、桔梗、蝉蜕各9克、谷精草、白蒺藜各15克。

2. 其他疗法

(1) 10%千里光眼液(89)，或10%黄连眼液滴眼(94)，每1至2小时1次。

(2) 银黄注射液(95)0.5毫升,球结膜下注射,每日1次。
(3) 滴扩瞳剂。
(4) 后期用退云散(98),每日1次。

9.2 单纯疱疹性角膜炎

单纯疱疹性角膜炎是常见的角膜病,近年来发病率显著增加。该病由热性疱疹病毒直接感染角膜上皮细胞所致。多为单眼患病,任何年龄均可罹患。相当于中医的聚星障。

病因病机

本病由外感风热之邪,内因肝火炽盛,内外合邪,上犯于目;或因饮食不节致脾胃湿热蕴积,而致发病;或因肝肾阴虚,虚火上炎。

临床表现

发病前常有上呼吸道感染发热史,自觉异物感,畏光流泪,视物不清,睫状充血,角膜浅层灰白色点状浸润,继而融合呈树枝状,浸润扩大加深,形成边缘不整齐的浅溃疡似地图状,角膜基质受累可并发虹膜炎。

辨证论治

1. 内治法

(1) 肝经风热

主证:有异物感,羞明流泪,角膜散在灰白色浸润点,伴有发热恶寒,舌苔薄黄,脉浮数。

治法:疏风清热。

方药:羌活胜风汤(42)。柴胡、荆芥、防风、前胡、羌活、独活、薄荷、川芎、白芷、黄芩、枳壳、桔梗各9克,白术12克,甘草6克。用法:水煎服,日1剂。

(2) 肝火炽盛

主证:眼部症状明显加重,视物模糊,角膜浸润扩大加深,兼头痛、尿赤、苔黄、脉弦数。

治法：清肝泻火。

方药：龙肝泻肝汤(40)加减。龙胆草、栀子、黄芩、柴胡、木通、泽泻各9克，生地黄15克，密蒙花30克，木贼草12克，赤芍15克。用法：水煎服，日1剂。

(3) 湿热蕴蒸

主证：角膜炎症经久不愈，头重胸闷，尿黄，大便稀，口粘，舌红苔黄腻，脉濡。

治法：化湿清热。

方药：三仁汤(8)加减。杏仁、薏苡仁、半夏、厚朴、竹叶、滑石各9克，金银花18克，蒲公英30克，蝉蜕9克，甘草6克。用法：水煎服，日1剂。

(4) 阴虚火旺

主证：角膜炎症较轻，但迁延不愈，舌红少苔，脉细数。

治法：滋阴清热。

方药：知柏地黄汤(43)加减。知母、黄柏、泽泻、山药各9克、茯苓、生地黄、草决明、谷精草各12克，玄参15克。用法：水煎服，日1剂。

2. 其他疗法

(1) 10%穿心莲眼液(96)，或10%千里光眼液(89)滴眼。

(2) 金银花、桑叶、野菊花、防风、蒲公英煎水，滤过后清洗眼，或作湿热敷。

(3) 病变后期用退云散(98)，以消除翳障。

(4) 针刺治疗：常用睛明、四白、承泣、丝竹空、合谷、光明、足三里等。每次取局部3穴，远端2穴，每日1次。

(5) 中成药：黄连上清丸(102)。

用法：每日两次，每次9克。

9.3 深层角膜炎

深层角膜炎是以角膜基质层有不规则浸润及水肿为特点。其病因可能由病毒感染，或某种过敏因素引起。中医称混睛障。

病因病机

多因肝经风热或热毒壅盛上攻于目；或邪毒久伏，耗损阴液，阴虚火旺所致。

临床表现

主觉轻微眼红，畏光流泪、眼痛，视物模糊，检查见睫状充血，角膜表层光滑，基质层呈灰白色毛玻璃样混浊，边界不清，也可呈边界清楚的圆盘状混浊，病变区角膜增厚，内皮水肿粗糙。本病可并发虹膜睫状体炎。

辨证论治

1. 内治法

(1) 风热壅盛

主证：羞明流泪，眼微痛，视物不清，睫状充血，角膜深层雾样混浊，兼头痛发热，舌红苔薄白或薄黄，脉浮数。

治法：疏风清热。

方药：桑菊饮(44)加减。桑叶、菊花、芦根、桔梗各12克，连翘、防风、薄荷、泽泻各9克、赤芍、茺蔚子各15克，甘草6克。用法：水煎服，日1剂。

加减。角膜水肿明显者加车前子12克，薏苡仁12克，炎症后期加决明子12克，白蒺藜12克。

(2) 肝脾湿热

主证：眼痛、羞明流泪加重，伴食欲不振，口臭、胸闷、便秘、舌红苔黄腻，脉数。

治法：清热化湿。

方药：银花解毒汤(45)加减。金银花30克，地丁15克，连翘9克，赤芍15克，夏枯草12克，生地黄15克，丹皮9克，藿香9克,半夏9克,厚朴9克。用法:水煎服,日1剂。

(3) 阴虚火旺

主证:眼部症状较轻,反复发作,舌红苔少,脉细数。

治法:滋阴降火。

方药:大补阴丸(46)加减。知母、黄柏、丹皮各9克,熟地、龟板、玄参各15克,密蒙花18克,木贼草12克,甘草6克。用法:水煎服,日1剂。

2. 其他疗法

(1)三黄眼液滴眼(97),每日4次。

(2)黄连西瓜霜眼液滴眼(88),每日3次。

(3)后期用犀黄散(91),每日3次。

(4)合并虹膜炎者用0.5%阿托品液,每日1次。

(5)中成药:羚翘解毒丸或黄连上清丸。每日2次,每次9克。

9.4 束状角膜炎

本病是以角膜表层粟粒疹并有一束新生血管伴随为特点,属过敏性角膜炎,多见于儿童,常反复发作,中医称风轮赤豆。

病因病机

多因肝经燥热致气血郁滞,或脾气虚弱,痰湿凝聚,痰气混结而致本病。

临床表现

初起在角膜缘有灰白色浸润点似泡疹,浸润渐向中心匐行,从角膜缘有一束新生血管伸入浸润之边缘,并随同向中心匐行,泡疹破溃成溃疡,痊愈后遗留圆形瘢痕性混浊,不同程度影响视力。主觉眼痛、异物感、流泪羞明,或有眼睑痉挛。

辨证论治

1. 内治法

(1) 肝经积热

主证：羞明流泪较重，异物感，眼痛，兼口苦咽干，舌红苔黄，脉弦数。

治法：泻肝清热。

方药：龙胆泻肝汤(40)加减。龙胆草、黄芩、栀子、柴胡、木通、泽泻各9克，生地黄、赤芍各15克，草决明、夏枯草各12克。用法：水煎服，日1剂。

(2) 脾虚挟痰

主证：眼部症状较轻，反复发作，伴面色苍白，四肢乏力，舌淡苔薄，脉弱。

治法：健脾益气，化痰散结。

方药：香贝养荣汤(47)加减。人参、白术、熟地、白芍、当归各12克，茯苓、川芎、桔梗、香附各9克，夏枯草、青葙子各12克。

2. 其他疗法

(1) 三黄眼液滴眼(97)，每日4至6次。

(2) 退云散(98)少许点眼，每日3次。

(3) 必要时可用抗菌素及激素滴眼。

9.5　角膜软化症

角膜软化症是以维生素A缺乏为主的高度营养不良引起的眼病。维生素A缺乏表现全身皮肤、粘膜、结膜及角膜出现干燥性变性，可导致失明。该病多见于儿童，均为双眼发病。中医称疳积上目。

病因病机

因饮食不节损伤脾胃，或喂养不当，或偏食，久病虚羸，致脾胃虚弱，脾失健运，酿成疳积；肝虚血少，目失所养，阴血不足，肝热内生也致本病。

临床表现

本病早期即出现夜盲，继而球结膜失去正常光泽，眼球向侧方转动时有皱褶,角膜暗淡无光,如病情继续加重则在睑裂部的球结膜出现三角形干燥斑,角膜呈毛玻璃样混浊,角膜上皮脱落,继发感染产生浸润、溃疡、前房积脓、溃疡穿孔、终致失明。

辨证论治

1.内治法

(1) 脾胃虚弱

主证:初起有夜盲,球结膜、角膜失去光泽,伴有腹胀,面黄消瘦,倦怠乏力,舌淡苔白稍厚,脉沉弱。

治法:益气健脾。

方药:参苓白术散(48)加减。党参12克,白术、茯苓、白芍、当归、山药、砂仁、陈皮、桔梗、扁豆各9克,甘草6克。用法:水煎服,日1剂。

(2) 脾虚肝热

主证:眼红、畏光流泪、角膜混浊,或有溃疡,兼腹胀便稀,午后潮热,烦躁不宁,苔浊腻,脉细濡或细而弦。

治法:健脾消疳,清肝泄热。

方药:肥儿丸(49)加减。党参12克,茯苓、白术、甘草、草决明、青葙子、芦荟、使君子各9克,山楂、神曲各12克,黄连6克,蒲公英18克。用法:水煎服,日1剂。

(3) 中焦虚寒

主证:角膜溃烂或穿孔,面色苍白,腹泻频繁,四肢不温。

治法:温阳散寒,补益脾胃。

方药:附子理中汤(50)加减。人参、白术、山药、附子、干姜各9克,熟地、黄芪、白芍各15克,陈皮、菊花各12克。用法:水煎服,日1剂。

2. 其他疗法

(1) 眼部用药可参考角膜溃疡。

(2) 口服或注射维生素AD。

(3) 针刺疗法:常选用中脘、足三里、胃俞、脾俞、肝俞等,每日1次,每次3至4穴。

(4) 推拿疗法以调理脾胃。

(5) 中成药:人参健脾丸(104),或十全大补丸(105),每日2次,每次服9克。

(蔡华松)

10 色素膜疾病

色素膜的血管十分丰富,对侵入人体的某些致敏物质或全身和局部炎症病灶,其反应特别灵敏,因此病因非常复杂。色素膜炎对视功能破坏严重,尤其是慢性炎症因发生合并症,终至失明,眼球萎缩。色素膜病在中医眼科属瞳神疾病。瞳神在五轮中属水轮,内应于肾,肝肾同源,故色素膜病多从肝肾辨证。其病因多为脏腑功能失调,或外感邪气所致,故在辨证治疗的同时还应查清病灶,针对病因治疗。

10.1 急性渗出性虹膜睫状体炎

本病主要表现在前葡萄膜,若炎症反复发作,或病情加重,可向后蔓延,演变为全色素膜炎,中医称瞳神紧小。

病因病机

多因肝经风热上犯于目;或湿热蕴蒸,上扰清窍,灼伤瞳仁;或由其他眼病累及而发病。

临床表现

起病急,自觉眼部疼痛,羞明流泪,视物模糊,检查可见睫状充血,或混合性充血,有睫状压痛,角膜内壁下方有灰白色或色素样渗出物附着,虹膜充血肿胀,纹理不清,房水混浊,严重者前房有纤维素性渗出,房水呈胶状。瞳孔缩小,光反应迟钝或消失,视力下降。

辨证论治

1. 内治法

(1) 肝经风热

主证:起病急,眼痛,畏光流泪,视物模糊,睫状充血,房水混浊，瞳孔小，兼头痛，口干咽燥，舌红，苔薄黄，脉浮数。

治法：疏风清热。

方药：新制柴连汤(39)加减。柴胡、黄连、黄芩、栀子、龙胆草、木通、荆芥、防风各9克，赤芍、蔓荆子、桑白皮各12克，甘草6克。用法：水煎服，日1剂。

(2) 湿热内蕴

主证：眼部症状加重，混合性充血，房水混浊，前房有纤维素样渗出物，口苦咽干，舌红苔黄腻，脉弦滑。

治法：清热利湿。

方药：抑阳酒连散(51)加减。独活、羌活、防己、白芷、防风、蔓荆子、黄芩、黄连、栀子、黄柏、知母、甘草各9克，生地15克。用法：水煎服，日1剂。

2. 其他疗法

(1) 散瞳剂滴眼，以防虹膜后粘连，缓解疼痛。

(2) 湿热敷，每日3次，每次半小时。

(3) 针刺疗法：常用穴位睛明、太阳、四白、丝竹空、合谷、足三里等，每次近端3穴，远端2穴，每日1次。

10.2 慢性色素膜炎

本症为全色素膜慢性炎症，多由急性炎症演变而来，相当于中医瞳神干缺。

病因病机

多因久病伤阴，阴虚火旺，虚火上炎；或脾肾阳虚，命门火衰，脉失濡养所致。

临床表现

轻者无何不适，仅视力逐渐减退。检查可见轻度睫状充血，角膜后壁少许沉着物，房水微混，虹膜纹理不清，瞳孔缘色素脱落，虹膜后粘连，或有Koeppe氏结节，瞳孔不圆似梅花样，玻璃体呈尘埃状或絮状混浊。病程较长者，出现虹膜环状后粘连、瞳孔闭锁、虹膜膨隆、周边虹膜前粘连、前房角粘连而导致眼压升高，此时主觉眼胀，头痛，视力明显减退。本病也因合并晶状体混浊，致视力丧失。慢性炎症未得到控制终致眼球萎缩，完全失明。

辨证论治

1. 内治法

(1) 阴虚火旺

主证：病情轻，病程长，并有反复发作，兼心烦不眠，五心烦热，舌干咽燥，舌红少苔，脉细数。

治法：滋阴降火

方药：知柏地黄汤(43)加减。盐知母、盐黄柏、丹皮、泽泻、茯苓各9克，生地黄、玄参、麦冬、赤芍各15克，甘草6克。用法：水煎服，日1剂。

(2) 脾肾阳虚

主证：眼部症状具备，兼形寒体冷，口泛清涎，舌淡苔白，脉沉。

治法：温补脾肾。

方药：附子理中汤(50)加减。附子、白术、干姜、炒栀子、黄芩各9克，党参、黄芪、白芍各15克。炙甘草9克。用法：水煎服，日1剂。

2. 其他疗法

(1) 局部用药同急性渗出性虹膜睫状体炎。

(2) 若继发青光眼，并发白内障可考虑手术治疗。

(3) 中成药 明目地黄丸(114)，或石斛夜光丸(109)，每日两次，每次9克。

(蔡华松)

11 晶状体疾病

晶状体疾病主要可分三类：(1)先天性晶状体异常；(2)晶状体位置改变；(3)晶状体混浊。晶状体皮质、核、囊膜的任何部位发生混浊称白内障。白内障可分先天性白内障和后天性白内障两大类。此将中医治疗效果较好的老年性白内障及外伤性白内障介绍如下。

11.1 老年性白内障

老年性白内障是后天性白内障中最常见的一种，系老年性退化的一种表现。属中医圆翳内障范畴。

病因病机

多因年老体衰，肝肾亏损，精血不足，气血虚弱不能上荣于目；或脾虚失运，精气不能上荣于目所致。

临床表现

早期自觉眼前有固定黑影，并常出现单眼复视，多视或屈光改变现象。由于晶状体混浊部位不同，视力障碍出现时间亦有不同。

1. 皮质性白内障是多见的类型，临床分为四期。

初发期：原瞳孔下晶状体透明，散瞳后可见晶状体赤道部有楔状混浊。此期发展缓慢，对视力无影响。

未熟期(膨胀期)：赤道部的楔状混浊逐渐向瞳孔区和深部发展，前房变浅。斜照法检查时，光线投照侧出现虹膜半月形投影，视力明显下降，此期晶状体膨胀，有青光眼素质的患者，有导致青光眼发作的可能。

成熟期：晶状体皮质呈灰白色全部混浊、虹膜投影消失，前房恢复正常，视力仅有光觉。

过熟期：内障成熟过久，混浊的皮质呈乳白色液化，钙化或有胆脂结晶，核下沉，上半部前房变深，可出现虹膜震颤。

2. 老年性核性白内障较少见，晶状体呈棕褐色或琥珀色混浊，呈黑色时称黑内障。皮质尚透明，视力下降明显，病程进展较缓慢，可持续数年而皮质不发生混浊。

辨证论治

本病病程较长，药物治疗适用于初发期，若晶状体混浊已明显时药物难以奏效，则采用手术治疗。

1. 内治法

(1) 肝肾两亏

主证：年老体衰，视物模糊，头昏耳鸣，腰膝酸软，舌淡脉细弱。

治法：补益肝肾

方药：杞菊地黄汤(52)。

熟地黄 24 克，山萸肉 12 克，干山药 12 克，泽泻 9 克，茯苓 9 克，丹皮 9 克，枸杞子 9 克，菊花 9 克，水煎服，1 日 1 剂。

(2) 脾气虚弱：

主证：视物昏花，精神萎靡，肢体倦怠，面色萎黄，食少便溏，舌淡苔白，脉缓或细弱。

治法：补脾益气

方药：益气聪明汤(53)

蔓荆子 12 克，黄芪 6 克，人参 6 克，黄柏 9 克，白芍药 9 克，炙甘草 3 克，葛根 3 克，水煎服，1 日 1 剂。

(3) 阴虚挟湿热

主证：目涩视昏，烦热口臭，口干不思饮，大便不畅，舌红苔黄腻。

治法：滋阴清热，宽中利湿。

方药：甘露饮(54)

生地9克，熟地9克，石斛9克，天门冬12克，麦门冬12克，黄芩9克，茵陈9克，甘草6克，枇杷叶24克。水煎服，1日1剂。

2. 其他疗法

(1) 常用中成药

石斛夜光丸(109)

用于肝肾两亏者，1次9克，1日3次，水冲服。

补中益气丸(115)

用于脾气虚弱者，1次18克，1日2次，水冲服。

(2) 针刺疗法：本法仍只适用于早期患者，且宜与内服药物配合使用。

常用穴：睛明、球后、攒竹、鱼腰、臂臑、合谷、足三里、三阴交，每日或隔日1次，每次2—3穴，8—10次为1疗程。

(3) 点药：法可林，白内停等滴眼，1日3次。

(4) 手术治疗：以上治疗无效时，待成熟期可手术治疗。

11.2 外伤性白内障

眼部钝挫伤，穿孔伤均可引起白内障。本病属中医惊震内障。

病因病机

多因眼部血络受伤，淤血停留，气血失和，络中滞结，渐致气结膏凝；或气血滞涩，脉络郁遏，精华不得上输，目失涵养，视觉略昏，日后渐重，结为内障。

临床表现

挫伤所致者，伤后晶状体前囊表面可见一细小的色素环，数周至数月自行消退，仅留囊下细小点状混浊或完全吸收，视力可不受影响。有时晶状体皮质可发生星芒状，树枝状或花冠状混浊，通常发展缓慢。

穿通伤所致者,可查见晶状体囊破口,有时破口封闭后晶状体仅局部混浊,且不发展。如破口大,房水浸入引起晶状体全部混浊,若混浊的皮质突入前房,可继发葡萄膜炎或青光眼。

辨证论治

1. 内治法

(1) 气血淤滞

主证:眼外伤者眼睑淤血肿胀,头疼眼痛,瞳孔略大,光反应迟钝,重者前房积血,晶状体微混浊,日久全混浊。

治法:和血行滞,除风止痛。

方药:除风益损汤(55)加减。

当归6克,白芍6克,熟地6克,川芎6克,藁本5克,前胡5克,防风5克,丹皮9克,生三七3克,红花6克,水煎服,1日1剂。

(2) 肝肾亏损:

主证:病后期,眼不红不肿,唯留部分内障形成。

治法:补益肝肾

方药:明目地黄汤(56)

熟地黄24克,山萸肉12克,山药12克,泽泻9克,茯神9克,丹皮9克,生地24克,柴胡12克,当归12克,五味子9克,水煎服,1日1剂。

2. 其他疗法

(1) 中成药:明目地黄丸(114)

用于后期内障形成时,1日2次,每次18克。

(2) 若内障形成时间较久方药难奏效时,光觉色觉尚好,可手术治疗。继发青光眼者也宜及早手术处理。

(王静波)

12 青光眼

青光眼是指眼内压升高，造成视功能损害的一种眼病。它分为原发性、先天性、继发性3类。前两类为双眼发病，继发性青光眼多为单眼。原发性青光眼又分开角型及闭角型两种。青光眼属中医瞳神疾病中五风内障，即绿风内障、青风内障、乌风内障、黑风内障、黄风内障，其中以绿风内障及青风内障多见，现介绍此两种青光眼如下。

12.1 急性闭角型青光眼

本病多见于老年女性，为双侧性，但可一眼先发病，两眼发作间隔时间不定，其发病多与情绪波动或过劳有关。起病急，以突然眼胀、眼红、视力骤降、伴恶心、呕吐为特征，中医称绿风内障。

病因病机

因情志不舒，肝气郁结，郁久化火，上犯于目；或因肝胆火炽，热极生风，风火攻目；或因痰湿内聚，郁久化火，痰火上扰；也可由过劳伤阴，阴虚阳亢，亢而生风，风阳上扰。

临床表现

根据发病过程分为四期。临床前期：当情绪波动后，有轻微头痛、眼胀、虹视、休息后可自行缓解。发作期：因眼压急剧升高而出现眼球胀痛，剧烈头痛，恶心呕吐，视力骤然下降。检查可见混合性充血，角膜水肿似毛玻璃样混浊，前房浅，虹膜呈扇形萎缩，瞳孔散大，光反应消失，晶状体前囊下灰白色混浊斑，前房角关闭。缓解期：经治疗后眼压下降，症状消退，视功能得到改善，充血消退，角膜透明，房角重新开放，但高眼压持续时间较长者，房角可形成粘连，此期长短不一。慢性期：急性发作未及时治疗，或反复发作前房角广泛粘连使眼压持续升高，视力显著减退，视野缩小，眼底视乳头杯盘比例增大，色淡，血管向鼻侧移位，呈屈膝状，房角变窄或关闭，渐渐视力全部丧失而进入绝对期。

辨证论治

1. 内治法

(1) 肝气郁结

主证：眼红眼胀痛、虹视、视力下降，有情志不舒、头痛、胸闷、恶心呕吐、舌红苔薄，脉弦细。

治法：疏肝理气，清热熄风。

方药：丹栀逍遥散(57)加减。柴胡、丹皮、栀子、白术、茯苓、甘草各9克，白芍、当归、半夏、白芷、菊花各12克，炒枣仁30克。用法：水煎服，日1剂。

(2) 肝胆火炽

主证：眼部症状具备，伴有恶心呕吐，恶寒发热，尿赤，便干，舌红苔黄，脉弦数。

治法：清肝泻火。

方药：绿风羚羊饮(58)加减。黄芩、知母、大黄、防风、泽泻、夏枯草各9克，玄参、茯苓、车前子各12克，羚羊角粉3克(冲服)。用法：水煎服，日1剂。

(3) 痰火上扰

主证：眼红胀痛，视物不清，头痛，恶心呕吐，动则眩晕，尿赤、便干，舌红苔黄腻，脉滑数。

治法：清热祛痰。

方药：半夏羚羊角散(59)加减。羚羊角薄荷、羌活、防风、半夏、川芎、泽泻、陈皮各9克，蔓荆子、菊花、决明子各12克、车前子15克。用法：水煎服，日1剂。

(4) 阴虚阳亢

主证：眼胀头痛，视物昏朦，心烦易怒，耳鸣耳聋，口干咽燥，舌红苔少，脉细数。

治法：滋阴清热

方药：羚羊钩藤饮(60)加减。钩藤、桑叶、菊花、茯苓各12克，生地、白芍各15克，半夏、竹茹、甘草各9克。羚羊角粉3克(冲服)。用法：水煎服，日1剂。

2. 其他疗法

(1) 2%槟榔液(99)、或1%丁公藤液(100)滴眼，每日3次。

(2) 针刺疗法常用穴位睛明、四白、承泣、球后、合谷、太冲、风池。每次主穴及配穴4处，每日1次。

(3) 耳针疗法，探查敏感点，再选配目$_1$、目$_2$、肝等穴，用耳针或贴压王不留行，直至症状缓解。

12.2 开角型青光眼

青风内障开角型青光眼是眼压升高，前房角为宽角，又称单纯性青光眼。本病进展缓慢，症状甚轻，不易早期发现。多见于青年人，男性多于女性，相当于中医青风内障。

病因病机

多因情志不舒，肝气郁结，郁而化火，上犯于目；或因脾虚湿困，湿而生痰，痰郁化火，痰火上扰；或因肝肾不足，真阴暗耗，虚火上炎。

临床表现

早期几乎无症状，当过劳或情绪波动时可出现轻微眼胀、头痛、虹视，随着病情进展，视力逐渐下降，视野日渐缩小，终至失明。检查眼前部无改变，眼底视乳头凹陷加大而深，杯盘比例超过0.5，血管向鼻侧移位，部分血管呈屈膝状，有神经纤维层缺损，晚期视乳头色苍白，呈杯状凹陷。前房角为宽角，眼压水平升高，24小时眼压波动幅度大。

辨证论治

1. 内治法

(1) 气郁化火

主证：有轻微眼胀，虹视，头痛，眩晕，胸胁胀满，舌红苔黄，脉弦细。

治法：清热疏肝。

方药：丹栀逍遥散(57)加减。柴胡、丹皮、栀子、茯苓、白术、白芷、菊花、夏枯草各9克，白芍、当归、勾藤各12克，羚羊角粉3克(冲服)。用法：水煎服，日1剂。

(2) 痰火相结

主证：眼部症状具备，兼头晕目眩，口苦咽燥，胸胁痞满，烦躁不宁，舌红苔黄腻，脉滑数。

治法：清热化痰。

方药：羚羊角散(61)加减。羚羊角粉3克，白菊花、决明子、蔓荆子、麦冬、茯神、赤芍、车前子各12克，竹茹、半夏、胆南星、甘草各9克。用法：水煎服，日1剂。

(3) 肝肾不足

主证：眼症具备，失眠健忘，腰膝酸软，头晕耳鸣，舌红少苔，脉细数。

治法：滋补肝肾。

方药：杞菊地黄汤(52)加减。枸杞、菊花、熟地、白芍、党参、茯神各12克，泽泻、车前子、天麻各9克。用法：水煎服，日1剂。

2. 其他疗法

(1) 1%丁公藤液滴眼，每日3次。

(2) 2%槟榔液滴眼，每日3次。

(3) 针刺治疗同急性闭角型青光眼。

(蔡华松)

13 眼底疾病

眼底病病种较多，本章将中药治疗效果较好的几种疾病介绍如下。

13.1 视网膜中央血管阻塞

包括视网膜中央动脉栓塞及中央静脉血栓，前者视力骤丧，后者视力下降较缓，部分病例可继发青光眼。本病属中医暴盲范畴。

病因病机

忿怒暴悖，肝气上逆，气血郁闭，脉络阻塞；或恣酒嗜辛，胃热蕴蒸，营气不从，血流阻滞；或劳思竭视，房劳过度，暗耗真阴，肝阳上越，上扰清窍；或脾失健运，痰湿停聚，兼气血不和，阳升风动，风痰相结，阻滞经络。

临床表现

病发突然，视力骤丧，或数日内迅速下降，但外眼正常。

眼底检查：视网膜中心动脉栓塞者，视网膜呈贫血现象，后极部视网膜呈灰白色混浊水肿，黄斑部表现樱桃红色，视乳头变白，境界模糊，压迫眼球时无动脉搏动，视网膜动脉显著变细，呈白线状；中心静脉血栓者，视神经乳头明显充血、水肿，边界模糊，视网膜水肿，静脉高度迂曲怒张，色紫红，有时隐藏于水肿的网膜组织内或混杂于出血斑中，呈节段状，动脉变细，视网膜及视神经乳头上有大量浅层火焰状、放射状和深层圆形出血斑，以及棉团状渗出物。出血量大时也可流入玻璃体内。日久视神经乳头表面和受累的静脉周围出现新生毛细血管网，可继发青光眼。

辨证论治

上两病能严重损伤视力，必须引起注意，在治疗上应针对病因，迅速采用中西两法进行急救，再根据病情缓急和病程长短，结合全身辨证予以治疗。

1. 内治法

(1) 气血郁闭

主证：发病之初视力骤丧，上述眼底变化悉具者。全身证见头晕头痛，胸胁胀痛，脉弦或弦涩。

治法：活血通窍。

方药：通窍活血汤(62)加味。

赤芍3克，川芎3克，桃仁9克(研泥)，红花9克，老葱3克，红枣7枚，麝香1.5克(后入)，郁金9克，青皮6克。加酒适量水煎服，1日1剂，睡前服。

加减：视网膜水肿甚者加琥珀6克，泽兰9克，益母草12克；眼底出血甚者加蒲黄12克，茜草12克，三七6克。

(2) 痰热上壅

主证：眼症同前，全身症有头眩而重，胸闷烦躁，食少恶心，痰稠口苦，舌苔黄腻，脉弦滑。

治法：涤痰开窍。

方药：涤痰汤(63)加味。

半夏8克(姜制)，胆星8克，橘红6克，枳实6克，茯苓6克，人参3克，菖蒲3克，竹茹2克，甘草2克，生姜6克，大枣7枚，僵蚕6克，地龙12克，川芎9克。水煎服，1日1剂。

(3) 肝风内动

主证：眼症同前，全身症见头晕耳鸣，面色潮红，烦躁易怒，失眠，口苦舌红，苔黄脉弦；或有腰膝酸软，遗精神疲，舌绛脉细。

治法：平肝潜阳，滋阴熄风。

方药：天麻钩藤饮(64)加味。

天麻9克，钩藤12克(后入)，石决明18克(先煎)，山栀9克，黄芩9克，川牛膝12克，杜仲9克，益母草9克，桑寄生9克，夜交藤9克，朱茯神9克，白芍12克，阿胶6克，丹参15克，地龙12克。水煎服，1日1剂。

2. 其他疗法

(1) 中成药：杞菊地黄丸(110)。用于本病后期，1日2次，1次18克。

(2) 视网膜中央动脉阻塞者，应立即用血管扩张剂急救，如亚硝酸异戊酯吸入，或硝酸甘油片舌下含化等。

(3) 针刺疗法：眶周穴位：睛明、球后、瞳子髎、承泣、攒竹、太阳等。远端穴位：风池、合谷、内关、外关、太冲、翳风、足光明、命门、肾俞等。每天选眶周穴位2个，远端穴位2个，轮流使用，只针不灸，不留针。

13.2 视网膜静脉周围炎

本病以视网膜出血和视网膜静脉的改变为特征，多发生于21—30岁男性青年，常双眼先后发病，易反复发作。属于中医的云雾移睛或暴盲范围。

病因病机

多为火热内扰，热伤营分，迫血妄行；或肝肾不足，虚火上炎，火郁脉络，气血逆乱；或心脾亏损，血虚气弱，失于统摄，而致血不循经溢于络外。

临床表现

病初起，视力无明显改变，偶见眼前少许黑影飘动，随病情变化可突然视力减退。

眼底表现：远端静脉迂曲扩张，血管旁有白鞘，周围有灰白色渗出及出血，出血可进入玻璃体，若大量出血则可致玻璃体高度混浊。大量、反复出血可形成视网膜和玻璃体内结缔组织增生，形成增殖性视网膜病变。

辨证论治

1. 内治法

(1) 火热上扰，迫血妄行

主证：视力骤降，眼底静脉充盈、怒张，出血量多而色鲜红，或玻璃体积血，眼底不辨，舌红苔黄，脉弦细数。

治法：清热泻火，凉血止血。

方药：宁血汤(69)。

仙鹤草12克，旱莲草12克，生地黄12克，栀子炭9克，白芍15克，白蔹9克，侧柏叶9克，阿胶6克，白茅根15克。水煎服，1日1剂。

加减：兼有烦躁易怒，口苦咽干加龙胆草9克，夏枯草12克。

(2) 阴虚火旺，火郁脉络

主证：反复出血但量较少，可伴少许新生血管，并见唇红颧赤，口苦咽干，眩晕耳鸣，腰酸遗精，五心烦热，舌绛苔少。

治法：滋阴降火。

方药：知柏地黄汤(43)。

熟地12克，山茱萸6克，山药6克，泽泻4.5克，茯苓4.5克，丹皮4.5克，知母30克，黄柏30克。水煎服，1日1剂。

(3) 心脾亏损，血虚气弱

主证：眼底血斑颜色较淡，而见面白神疲，怠惰懒言，心悸怔忡，纳呆便溏，舌淡脉虚者。

治法：养心健脾，益气明目。

方药：归脾汤(82)。

白术30克，茯神30克，黄芪30克，桂圆肉30克，酸枣仁30克，人参15克，木香15克，炙甘草8克，当归3克，远志3克(蜜炙)，生姜6克，大枣7枚。水煎服，1日1剂。

(4) 瘀血滞结

主证：病情顽固，久治而视力改善不明显，眼底血斑暗红，或有结缔组织增殖，舌色紫暗或有淤斑者。

治法：活血祛淤，软坚散结。

方药：祛淤汤(70)。

生地15克，旱莲草15克，仙鹤草12克，桃仁9克，赤芍9克，泽兰12克，丹参15克，川芎9克，郁金12克，当归9克。水煎服，1日1剂。

2. 其他疗法

(1) 用田三七或红花溶液作离子导入。

(2) 玻璃体出血较多时，经以上治疗3—6个月无好转者，可施行玻璃体切割术。

13.3 中心性浆液性脉络膜视网膜病变

本病以眼底黄斑区水肿，视物变形为特点，有视物模糊，好发于中年男性，多为单眼发病，少数为双眼先后得病，易反复发作。属于中医视瞻昏渺范畴。

病因病机

脾失健运，致精微不化，不能运精于目；或痰湿困阻中焦，湿热蕴蒸，蒙蔽清窍；或情志郁结，玄府阻闭，以致气滞血淤；或肝肾不足，精血耗损，目失涵养；或心营亏损，神光虚耗，或用目不当，气血暗耗，以致神光涣散。

临床表现

早期眼前出现暗影，随之中心视力减退，注视区中心有固定的暗影。有视物变小或变形，并可伴有视物变色。

眼底检查：黄斑区呈灰红色或灰白色盘状水肿，其边缘有圆形或卵圆形的反光轮，中心凹反射消失。继之黄斑区出现黄白色点状渗出物。恢复期水肿或渗出物逐渐吸收，黄斑区遗留色素紊乱，中心凹反射重现，视力逐渐恢复。

眼底血管荧光造影检查，在黄斑水肿区可见荧光渗漏现象。

辨证论治

1. 内治法

(1) 浊邪上犯

主证：自觉视物昏矇，视物变形。眼底可见黄斑区水肿、黄白色渗出点，中心凹反光消失，病情常缠绵不愈。伴有头重胸闷，食少口苦，尿黄少，舌苔黄腻，脉濡数。

治法：利湿清热，祛痰化湿。

方药：三仁汤(7)。

杏仁15克，滑石18克，白通草6克，白蔻仁6克，竹叶6克，厚朴6克，生薏仁18克，半夏6克。水煎服，1日1剂。

加减：黄斑区水肿明显者可选加茺蔚子12克，泽泻9克，车前子12克；若渗出物较多者可选加竹茹12克，胆星6克，枳实6克。

(2) 气滞血郁

主证：眼部症状同前，兼有情志不舒，头晕胁痛，口苦咽干，脉弦细数。

治法：清热疏肝，行气活血。

方药：丹栀逍遥散(57)。

柴胡15克，当归15克，白芍15克，白术15克，茯苓15克，甘草3克，生姜2片，薄荷3克，丹皮3克，栀子3克。水煎服，1日1剂。

(3) 肝肾不足

主证：眼内干涩，视物模糊，黄斑区水肿轻，有轻微色素沉着。兼有头晕耳鸣，失眠多梦，腰膝酸软，舌淡少苔，脉细。

治法：补益肝肾。

方药：加减驻景丸(65)。

菟丝子12克，褚实子12克，茺蔚子9克，枸杞子6克，车前子6克，木瓜6克，寒水石6克，紫河车粉9克(冲服)，生三七粉1.5克(冲服)，五味子6克。水煎服，1日1剂。

(4) 心脾两虚

主证：视力恢复缓慢，眼底水肿及渗出物较轻，但消退较难，兼见面色无华，头晕心悸，食少神疲，舌淡脉弱。

治法：养心益脾，补血行血。

方药：人参养荣汤(66)。

白芍 30 克，当归 10 克，陈皮 10 克，黄芪 10 克，肉桂 10 克，人参 10 克，白术 10 克，炙甘草 10 克，熟地 9 克，五味子 9 克，茯苓 9 克，炒远志 6 克，生姜 3 片，大枣 2 枚。水煎服，1 日 1 剂。

2. 其他疗法

针灸疗法：常用穴位，睛明、球后、头临泣、太阳、风池、翳明、合谷、养老、光明、肝俞、肾俞、足三里等。每次局部取 2 穴，远端配 2 穴，每日针 1 次，10 次为 1 疗程。

13.4　视网膜色素变性

视网膜色素变性是慢性进行性疾病，均为双眼发病，有明显的家族遗传因素。男性多见。本病属于中医的高风内障。

病因病机

禀赋不足，命门火衰；或肝肾亏损，精血不足；或脾胃虚弱，清阳不升等原因均可使脉道不得充盈，血流滞涩，目失所养。

临床表现

双眼受累，夜盲，早期白天视力不受影响，久之视力渐退，视野初期为环形暗点，逐渐向心性缩小呈管状终至失明。眼底见视网膜动脉和静脉高度狭窄，视神经乳头呈蜡黄或黄白色，以及骨细胞样的视网膜色素沉着。后期可并发白内障和青光眼。

辨证论治

(1) 命门火衰

主证：眼症如上，形寒肢冷，腰膝酸软，夜尿频繁，舌淡脉沉弱。

治法：温补肾阳。

方药：右归丸(67)。

熟地 24 克，山药 12 克，山茱萸 9 克，枸杞子 12 克，鹿角胶 12 克，菟丝子 12 克，杜仲 12 克，当归 9 克，肉桂 12 克，制附子 6 克。水煎服，1 日 1 剂。

(2) 肝肾两亏

主证：除以上眼症外，眼内干涩不适，头晕耳鸣，失眠多梦，舌红少苔，脉细数。

治法：滋养肝肾。

方药：明目地黄汤(56)加味。

熟地黄 24 克，山茱萸 12 克，山药 12 克，泽泻 9 克，茯神 9 克，丹皮 9 克，生地 24 克，柴胡 9 克，当归 9 克，五味子 6 克，丹参 18 克，牛膝 12 克，夜明砂 9 克，毛冬青 12 克。水煎服，1 日 1 剂。

(3) 脾气虚弱

主证：眼部症状如上，兼面白神疲，食少乏力，舌淡苔薄脉弱。

治法：补脾益气。

方药：补中益气汤(16)。

黄芪 15 克，甘草 5 克，人参 10 克，当归 10 克，橘皮 6 克，升麻 3 克，柴胡 3 克，白术 10 克。水煎服，1 日 1 剂。

2. 其他疗法

针刺疗法：取睛明、球后、承泣、瞳子髎、攒竹、肝俞、肾俞、脾俞、足三里、三阴交等，每次选 3—4 穴，每日或隔日 1 次，10 次为 1 疗程。

耳针取目$_1$、目$_2$、肝、心、肾、胆每次取穴 3 个，留针 30 分钟以上，或以上耳穴压豆。

13.5 视神经炎

视神经炎根据发病部位不同分为视神经乳头炎及球后视神经炎。本病多见于青壮年，多为双眼发病。

病因病机

本病多因情志郁结，肝失条达，气郁络阻；或肝胆火旺，上扰清窍；或肝肾阴虚，虚火上炎；或产后哺乳，气血虚衰。

临床表现

视神经乳头炎起病急，视力迅速减退至失明。眼底检查可见乳头充血水肿，境界模糊，生理凹陷消失，轻度隆起，周围视网膜水肿混浊，有少量火焰状出血及灰白色软性渗出斑。视网膜中央静脉充盈迂曲。

急性球后视神经炎，视力急剧下降，甚至光感消失。球后压痛，瞳孔光反应不持久。眼底检查早期无改变，或只有在病变接近视神经乳头时，才能见到视乳头轻度充血和边缘稍模糊。静脉充盈，后期视乳头色泽变淡或苍白。有哑铃样暗点。

慢性球后视神经炎视力缓降。早期眼底无改变，后期出现视神经萎缩。有中心或旁中心暗点。

辨证论治

1. 内治法

(1) 肝气郁结

主证：以上眼症之一，兼见平素情志抑郁，出现头晕目眩，胁痛，口苦咽干，胸闷不舒。

治法：疏肝解郁。

方药：逍遥散(83)。

柴胡15克，当归15克，白芍15克，白术15克，茯苓15克，甘草3克，生姜2片，薄荷3克。水煎服，1日1剂。

(2) 肝胆火盛

主证：单眼或双眼发病，视力急降，甚至失明，兼头痛眩晕，面红目赤，胁痛口苦，溺黄，舌边尖红，苔黄腻，脉弦数者。

治法：泻肝清火。

方药：龙胆泻肝汤(40)。

龙胆草6克，黄芩9克，栀子9克，泽泻12克，木通9克，车前子9克，当归3克，生地黄9克，柴胡6克，甘草6克。水煎服，1日1剂。

(3) 阴虚火旺

主证：眼症同前，兼头晕目眩，耳鸣、耳聋，唇红颧赤，舌质红，脉弦细数者。

治法：滋阴降火。

方药：知柏地黄汤(43)。

熟地黄24克，山茱萸12克，干山药12克，泽泻9克，茯苓9克，丹皮9克，知母30克，黄柏30克。水煎服，1日1剂。

(4) 气血虚弱

主证：病程后期，炎症已缓解，视神经乳头色泽稍淡。面色萎黄，消瘦，精神困倦，舌淡苔薄脉弱。

治法：调补气血。

方药：八珍汤(68)。

当归10克，川芎5克，白芍药8克，熟地黄15克，人参3克，炒白术10克，茯苓8克，甘草5克，生姜3片，大枣2枚。水煎服，1日1剂。

2. 其他疗法

(1) 以上各类型在病情稍缓后可酌情分别用逍遥丸(111)、龙胆泻肝丸(112)、知柏地黄丸(113)、十全大补丸(105)等中成药。

(2) 针刺疗法：可配合其他疗法应用。

常用穴：睛明、球后、攒竹、鱼腰、丝竹空、风池、三阴交、内关。

(3) 急性期可配合用激素,能较快控制病情进展。

(王静波)

14 玻璃体疾病

玻璃体呈无色透明胶体状，充满玻璃体腔，它易受视网膜、脉络膜病变的影响而发生混浊，眼外伤及玻璃体退行性变也可引起混浊、液化、后脱离等，导致视力减退，甚至失明。玻璃体中医称神膏，也属瞳神范畴。故发病也多责之于肝肾。

14.1 玻璃体混浊

玻璃体混浊可由眼内炎症、出血及退行性产物造成，它主要表现为眼前黑影飘动，视物不清，中医称云雾移睛。

病因病机

因湿热蕴蒸，浊气上犯；或因肝气郁结，致气滞血瘀血溢脉外；或因肝肾亏损，虚心上炎。

临床表现

轻症眼前有黑影飘舞似飞蚊样，视力多数无变化；重症眼前似有膜样物遮盖，视力减退，甚至失明。检查外眼无异常，玻璃体有尘埃状、或絮状，或团块状混浊，混浊物可呈灰黄色，或呈红色。因混浊程度不同，眼底检查清晰可见，或模糊窥及，或完全不能见。

辨证论治

首先应查明导致玻璃体混浊的原因，针对病因治疗。

1. 内治法

(1) 湿热蕴蒸

主证：眼前黑影飘荡，视物模糊，玻璃体混浊，伴头重、胸闷、口苦，舌苔黄腻，脉濡数。

治法：清热利湿。

方药：三仁汤(8)加减。杏仁、薏苡仁、白蔻仁、通草、淡竹叶、厚朴、半夏各9克，滑石12克，赤芍15克。加减：湿重者加车前子、泽泻各9克。热重者加黄芩、栀子各9克、金银花24克。用法：水煎服，日1剂。

(2) 气滞血瘀

主证：视物不清或看不见，玻璃体积血呈尘埃状或团块状，伴情志不舒，胸闷胁胀，口苦舌质暗红有瘀斑，苔白或微黄，脉弦紧或涩。

治法：疏肝理气，止血祛瘀。

方药：丹栀逍遥散(57)加减。丹皮、栀子、柴胡、白术各9克，当归、赤芍、茯苓各12克。

加减：新鲜出血加仙鹤草、旱莲草、生蒲黄各12克，三七粉3克(冲服)。陈旧积血加桃仁、红花、川芎、枳壳各9克，郁金、茺蔚子各12克。用法：水煎服，日1剂。

(3) 阴虚火旺

主证：视物模糊，眼前黑影飘动，头晕耳鸣，腰膝酸软，口干咽燥，舌红少苔，脉细数。

治法：滋阴降火。

方药：知柏地黄汤(43)加减。盐知母、盐黄柏、生地黄、丹皮、泽泻、茯苓各9克，牛膝12克，赤芍、麦冬各15克，丹参18克，甘草6克。用法：水煎服，日1剂。

2. 其他疗法

用丹参、或三七、或红花注射液作电离子透入。

(蔡华松)

15 眼眶疾病

眼眶疾病病因较多，中医药对部分眶内炎症性病变疗效较好，本章就临床上治疗效果较好的部分眶内疾病介绍如下。

15.1 眼眶急性炎症

一般发病较急，眼球胀痛突起，多见于眶骨骨膜炎，眶蜂窝组织炎，眼球筋膜炎等疾病。属于中医的突起睛高症。

病因病机

多因内热火毒上冲于眼或因兼挟痰饮，渍于脏腑，蕴积生热，热冲于目；或因五脏毒风所蕴，热极充目，毒攻五轮。

临床表现

起病急速，不同程度眼球突出，眼睑皮肤红肿，结膜充血，水肿，可伴眼球运动受限或完全固定，剧烈眼痛头痛，甚者全身出现高烧，恶心，呕吐，可继发为全眼球炎，脑膜炎，海绵窦血栓性静脉炎的危险。

辨证论治

1. 内治法

(1) 热毒壅滞

主证：眼症同上，病情初起，兼发热恶寒，舌红苔黄，脉数或浮数等。

治法：清火解毒，活血消肿。

方药：仙方活命饮(71)五味消毒饮(5)加减。

前方中穿山甲3克，天花粉3克，甘草节3克，乳香3克，白芷3克，赤芍3克，贝母3克，防风3克，没药3克，皂角刺3克，归尾3克，陈皮9克，金银花9克。后方中野菊花6克，蒲公英6克，紫花地丁6克，紫背天葵6克。水煎服，1日1剂。

(2) 热毒入里

主证：眼症同上较重，头眼剧痛，兼壮热烦渴，面赤气粗，溲黄便秘，舌质红绛，脉数有力等症。

治法：清营解毒。

方药：清营汤(4)加减。

犀角2克，生地黄15克，元参9克，竹叶心3克，麦冬9克，丹参6克，黄连5克，金银花9克，连翘6克，水煎服，1日1剂。

2. 其他疗法

(1) 外治可用葱，艾捣烂炒热布包以温熨。

(2) 白芷、细辛、当归、苍术、麻黄、防风、羌活煎汤熏洗。

(3) 若有脓者可切开排脓。

(4) 病情较急重者，可配合用抗菌素。

15.2 眼眶假性肿瘤

是一种非特异性慢性增殖性炎症，原因不明，能引起眼球突出及眼球运动障碍，多为单眼发病，男性多于女性。本病应与真性肿瘤相鉴别。属于中医的鹘眼凝睛症。

病因病机

风热毒邪上壅头目，眼络滞涩，气血淤阻；或邪热亢盛，日久伤阴，阴液亏耗，血运滞涩，气血淤滞所致。

临床表现

眼球突出，眼球运动障碍，约半数患者有炎症表现，眼痛，结膜充血，水肿，多数患者可触及边界不清，固定的肿物，有压痛，严重时眶内可被肿块充满，早期视力和眼底多无变化，极少数晚期病例中可见到眼后极部受压现象。

辨证论治

1. 内治法

(1) 风热毒邪壅盛，眼络淤阻：

主证：眼球突起，球结膜充血，运动受限，伴头痛项强，面红身热等全身症状。舌红苔黄，脉数。

治法：祛风清热解毒，活血通络。

方药：泻脑汤(72)加减：

黄芩9克，大黄6克，元明粉3克，车前子9克，木通6克，茯苓9克，防风6克，桔梗9克，茺蔚子12克，元参12克，黄连6克，赤芍12克，当归12克。水煎服，1日1剂。

(2) 邪热亢盛，日久阴虚血淤

主证：眼症同上，全身可伴有头晕耳鸣，五心烦热，心悸失眠，形体消瘦，舌暗红，脉弦细而涩等。

治法：滋阴清热，化淤散结。

方药：通幽汤(73)加减

熟地黄9克，炙甘草3克，当归6克，红花3克，桃仁12克，生地黄9克，女贞子12克，旱莲草15克，龟板12克，鳖甲12克，夏枯草15克，牡蛎15克。水煎服，1日1剂。

2. 其他疗法

(1) 可配合应用抗菌素及激素治疗。

(2) 对以淋巴细胞增生为主者，适用放射治疗。

(3) 可用三棱针刺迎香、太阳、上星及上睑出血，开涩导滞，泻其有余。

(王静波)

16 眼肌疾病

斜视是指两眼相对位置不正常,造成双眼视觉紊乱的主要原因,它包括共同性斜视与非共同性斜视两种。斜视眼因长期受到抑制而形成弱视。

16.1 麻痹性斜视

本病有先天性及后天性两种,前者为先天发育异常,以手术治疗为主。本节仅讨论后天性麻痹性斜视,它是以神经或肌肉损害致眼球运动受限,眼位偏斜,复视为特点,中医称风牵偏视。

病因病机

多因正气不足,卫外失固,风热乘虚而入,直中脉络;或因脾失健运,聚湿生痰,复感风邪,风痰阻络;或因气血虚弱,筋络失养。

临床表现

起病猝然,眼位偏斜,运动受限,多为单眼发病。双眼视突然受破坏而出现复视、眩晕、恶心或呕吐。经过一阶段后麻痹眼完全恢复正常,或形成单眼抑制,复视可消失。

辨证论治

1. 内治法

(1) 风邪中络

主证:眼球突然偏斜,运动受限,复视、头痛,恶寒发热,苔薄白,脉浮。

治法:疏风通络。

方药:小续命汤(74)加减。麻黄、防风、防己、附子、川芎、生姜各9克,白芍、党参、葛根各15克。黄芩、甘草各6

克。用法：水煎服，日1剂。

(2) 风痰阻络

主证：眼部表现同前，兼食欲不振，痰多，舌苔厚腻，脉弦滑。

治法：健脾化痰，祛风通络。

方药：六君子汤(75)合正容汤(76)。茯苓、白术、半夏、白附子、僵蚕、羌活、防风各9克，赤芍、党参、勾藤各15克，甘草6克。用法：水煎服，日1剂。

(3) 气血不足

主证：眼部症状具备，兼半身不遂，面色萎黄，舌质淡，苔白，脉细。

治法：益气养血。

方药：补阳还五汤(77)加减。桃仁、红花、川芎、归尾、白附子、僵蚕、葛根各9克，黄芪、赤芍、石决明、地龙各15克。用法：水煎服，日1剂。

2. 其他疗法

(1) 针刺疗法　常用瞳子髎、承泣、颊车、地仓、太阳、牵正、合谷、太冲等，每次局部三穴，远端二穴，每日1次。

(2) 灸法　在上述局部穴处用火灸。

(3) 维生素B_1及维生素B_{12}等肌肉注射。

16.2　共同性斜视

共同性斜视是眼位偏斜，眼球无论往何方向转动斜度不变，中医称小儿通睛。

病因病机

小儿体稚，筋络脆嫩，遇风热攻损，经络凝滞而发病，或因恐吓、外伤等致气血凝滞，筋脉受损。

临床表现

发病多在三岁左右，眼球可向水平或垂直方向偏位，以前者多见,眼球运动无障碍,向各方位运动,斜视角不变,斜视眼因长期受抑制而无复视,并形成弱视,若为交替性斜视则不形成弱视。

辨证论治

本症早期治疗效果较好,若斜视眼已形成弱视,则以滋补肝肾,益气养血为主。

1. 内治法

(1) 风热攻目,经络凝滞,宜祛风清热,活血通络。

方药:龙胆泻肝汤(40)合桃红四物汤(78)。龙胆草、黄芩、栀子、柴胡、车前子各9克,生地黄、当归、赤芍各15克。制桃仁、红花各6克。用法:水煎服,日1剂。

(2) 惊恐致气滞血凝,宜安神镇惊,活血养血。

方药:安神镇惊丸(116)加减。党参、茯神、麦冬、当归、薄荷、黄连、栀子各9克,生地黄、赤芍各15克,炒枣仁30克,柏子仁18克。用法:水煎服,日1剂。

(3) 外伤致筋脉受损,宜活血行淤,化痰通络。

方药:通血丸(79)加减。荆芥、防风、羌活、藁本、川芎、陈皮、半夏、胆南星各9克,赤芍、当归、生地黄各15克。用法:水煎服,日1剂。

2. 其他疗法

(1) 药物治疗效果不好者,应及早手术治疗。

(2) 斜眼弱视较重者,可配合弱视训练。

(蔡华松)

17 眼外伤

眼外伤是指眼球及其附属器由于意外而引起的损伤，本章着重讨论眼挫伤及穿孔伤。

17.1 眼挫伤

眼挫伤是指眼部受钝器的冲击而引起的一系列眼部损伤。属中医眼科的撞击伤目范畴。

病因病机

常因撞碰、球击、木头、石块、砖瓦、皮带、棍棒、铁块等物的钝力打击，撞伤眼睑或眼球内各部分组织。

临床表现

挫伤后轻者可引起眼睑水肿，皮下淤血，结膜水肿，充血，角膜擦伤，上皮脱落，重者可引起眼球裂伤或前房积血，虹膜根部断离，瞳孔散大，晶状体脱位，玻璃体积血，脉络膜破裂，视网膜震荡，出血，脱离，黄斑部渗出，水肿等。

辨证论治

1. 内治法

(1) 络伤出血

主证：眼睑青肿，重坠难睁，或眶内淤血，眼球突出；或白睛溢血，或血灌瞳神，或眼底出血。

治法：止血为先，活血为后。

方药：十灰散(80)加减。

大蓟、小蓟、荷叶、侧柏叶、茅根、茜草、山栀、大黄、牡丹皮、棕榈皮以上药各等份，烧灰存性，研极细末，白藕捣汁，调服，每次15克，食后服下。

出血静止改用活血化淤法，用祛淤汤(70)

归尾12克，赤芍12克，桃仁9克，泽兰9克，丹参15克，川芎6克，郁金12克，生地12克，旱莲草12克，仙鹤草12克。水煎服，1日1剂。

(2) 气滞血淤

主证：昏矇，检查见晶状体混浊，玻璃体混浊，视网膜水肿，眼睛刺痛或胀痛等。

治法：行气活血，化淤止痛。

方药：桃红四物汤(78)加减。

熟地黄15克，川芎9克，白芍药12克，当归12克，桃仁6克，红花6克，丹皮12克，丹参15克，郁金12克，枳壳6克。水煎服，1日1剂。

2. 其他疗法

(1) 中成药：杞菊地黄丸(110)。

用于病的后期以提高视力。1日2次，1次18克。

(2) 有前房积血及玻璃体积血较重者，眼垫封盖双眼，卧床休息。配合三七或丹参离子透入。

(3) 有裂伤及内容物脱出者应修复伤口，预防感染。

17.2 眼球穿通伤

为由于锐器刺伤或细小金属矿石碎片，爆炸弹片，崩溅入眼所造成，病情与损伤的部位，原因，程度，有无异物存留或感染有关。属中医眼科的真睛破损。

病因病机

眼球被刀、剪、锥、针等锐利之物戳破；或高速飞溅之金属碎屑，或爆炸之破片，碎石飞射入眼。

临床表现

受伤眼可有不同程度的疼痛，羞明，流泪，眼睑疼挛及视力障碍等症状。可造成黑睛全层破裂或白睛裂伤。症见房水外溢，前房变浅或消失，前房积血，瞳仁不圆，晶状体脱位或破裂；甚者导致眼内容物绽出，最终眼球变形而失明。

眼球穿通伤后，应注意观察有无继发感染，球内异物遗留及交感性眼炎的发生。

辨证论治

1. 内治法

(1) 气滞血瘀

主证：眼组织损伤，眼球疼痛，眼红羞明流泪。

治法：活血化瘀祛风。

方药：除风益损汤(55)。

当归6克，白芍6克，熟地6克，川芎6克，藁本5克，前胡5克，防风5克。

加减：角膜混浊者加木贼6克，菊花9克，蝉蜕9克；眼底水肿时加泽泻12克，车前子9克，茯苓9克；畏光流泪加羌活6克，薄荷6克，龙胆草9克；痛甚者加乳香6克，没药6克。水煎服，1日1剂。

(2) 络伤出血

主证：见白睛溢血，或血灌瞳神，或眼底出血。

治法：凉血止血。

方药：十灰散(80)。

大蓟、小蓟、荷叶、侧柏叶、茅根、茜草、山栀大黄、牡丹皮、棕榈皮以上药各等份，烧灰存性，研极细末白藕捣汁，调服，每次15克，食后服下。

(3) 邪毒炽盛

主证：眼痛甚，创口肿胀，前房积脓，甚或全眼球炎。

治法：清热解毒，凉血活血。

方药：五味消毒饮(5)合犀角地黄汤(81)。

金银花9克，野菊花6克，蒲公英6克，紫花地丁6克，紫背天葵6克，犀角3克，生地黄30克，芍药12克，牡丹皮9

克。水煎服，1日1剂。

2. 其他疗法

(1) 及早清创缝合，并清除异物，预防感染。

(2) 视病情而定，注射破伤风抗毒素，以预防破伤风。

(3) 局部0.5%阿托品液散瞳，0.5%考的松及抗菌素眼药水点眼。

(王静波)

附 篇

(1)银翘散《温病条辨》

金银花 连翘 桔梗 薄荷 淡竹叶 荆芥穗 甘草 淡豆豉 牛蒡子 芦根

(2)内疏黄连汤《医宗金鉴》

栀子 连翘 薄荷 甘草 黄芩 黄连 桔梗 大黄 当归 白芍 木香 槟榔

(3)普济消毒饮《目经大成》

黄芩 黄连 陈皮 甘草 玄参 连翘 板蓝根 马勃 牛蒡子 薄荷 柴胡 僵蚕 升麻 桔梗

(4)清营汤《温病条辨》

犀角 玄参 麦冬 金银花 生地黄 丹参 连翘 黄连 竹叶卷心

(5)五味消毒饮《医宗金鉴》

金银花 野菊花 蒲公英 紫花地丁 紫背天葵

(6)散热消毒饮子《审视瑶函》

黄连 黄芩 连翘 牛蒡子 薄荷 羌活 防风

(7)黄连解毒汤《外台秘要》

黄芩 黄连 黄柏 栀子

(8)三仁汤《温病条辨》
杏仁　滑石　通草　淡竹叶　厚朴　薏苡仁　半夏　白蔻仁

(9)除湿汤《眼科纂要》
连翘　滑石　车前子　枳壳　黄芩　黄连　木通　甘草　陈皮　荆芥　茯苓　防风

(10)加减四物汤《审视瑶函》
苦参　薄荷　川芎　生地黄　牛蒡子　连翘　花粉　防风　赤芍　当归　荆芥穗

(11)化坚二陈皮《医宗金鉴》
陈皮　制半夏　茯苓　生甘草　白僵蚕　黄连

(12)防风散结汤《目经大成》
荆芥　防风　独活　红花　苏木　当归　石斛　蒲黄　滑石　桑白皮　蚕砂　土茯苓　白芍药

(13)燥湿汤《审视瑶函》
黄连　苍术　白术　陈皮　茯苓　半夏　枳壳　栀子　甘草

(14)柴胡散《审视瑶函》
柴胡　防风　赤芍　荆芥　羌活　桔梗　生地黄　甘草

(15)黄芪汤《秘传眼科龙木论》
黄芪　茺蔚子　防风　地骨皮　茯苓　大黄　人参　黄芩　甘草

(16)补中益气汤《东垣十书》
黄芪　炙甘草　党参　当归　陈皮　升麻　柴胡　白术

(17)助阳活血汤《证治准绳》
黄芪 炙甘草 防风 当归 白芷 蔓荆子 升麻 柴胡

(18)肾气丸《金匮要略》
熟地黄 山药 山萸肉 丹皮 泽泻 茯苓 炮附子 肉桂

(19)止泪补肝散《医宗金鉴》
当归 熟地黄 川芎 白芍 白蒺藜 木贼草 防风

(20)泻脾除热饮《银海精微》
黄芪 防风 茺蔚子 桔梗 大黄 黄芩 黄连 车前子 芒硝

(21)千金托里散《眼科集成》
党参 生黄芪 茯苓 甘草 当归 白芍药 川芎 桔梗 银花 白芷 防风 麦冬

(22)竹叶泻经汤《原机启微》
柴胡 栀子 羌活 升麻 炙甘草 黄芩 黄连 大黄 茯苓 赤芍药 泽泻 草决明 车前子 竹叶

(23)除风清脾饮《审视瑶函》
陈皮 连翘 防风 知母 玄明粉 黄芩 玄参 黄连 荆芥穗 大黄 桔梗 生地黄

(24)清脾凉血汤《医宗金鉴》
陈皮 苍术 白藓皮 厚朴 赤芍药 大黄 连翘 蝉蜕 荆芥 防风 竹叶 生甘草 玄参

(25)归芍红花散《审视瑶函》

当归 大黄 栀子 黄芩 红花 赤芍药 甘草 白芷 防风 连翘 生地黄

(26)驱风散热饮子《审视瑶函》

连翘 牛蒡子 羌活 薄荷 大黄 赤芍药 防风 当归尾 甘草 栀子 川芎

(27)泻肺饮《眼科纂要》

石膏 赤芍药 黄芩 桑白皮 枳壳 木通 连翘 荆芥 防风 栀子 白芷 羌活 甘草

(28)清肝散《审视瑶函》

当归尾 川芎 薄荷 生地黄 羌活 栀子 大黄 龙胆草 防风 甘草

(29)清瘟败毒饮《疫疹一得》

石膏 生地黄 犀角 黄连 黄芩 栀子 桔梗 知母 赤芍药 连翘 玄参 甘草 丹皮 竹叶

(30)桑白皮汤《审视瑶函》

桑白皮 泽泻 玄参 甘草 麦门冬 黄芩 旋复花 菊花 地骨皮 桔梗 茯苓

(31)泻肺汤《审视瑶函》

桑白皮 黄芩 地骨皮 知母 麦门冬 桔梗

(32)清燥救肺汤《医门法律》

冬桑叶 石膏 火麻仁 麦门冬 阿胶 枇杷叶 杏仁 党参 甘草

(33)冶金汤《目经大成》

玄参 桑白皮 枳壳 黄连 杏仁 旋复花 防风 黄芩 菊花 葶苈子

(34)消风除热汤《眼科集成》

柴胡 前胡 荆芥 防风 白芷 薄荷 胆草 大黄 葛根 石膏 甘草 黄芩

(35)当归活血饮《审视瑶函》

当归 熟地黄 白芍药 川芎 羌活 薄荷 黄芪 防风 苍术 甘草

(36)泻心汤《眼科纂要》

黄连 生地黄 连翘 赤芍药 当归尾 车前子 荆芥 防风 枳壳 甘草 石膏

(37)滋阴降火汤《审视瑶函》

生地黄 麦门冬 知母 黄柏 黄芩 当归 川芎 熟地黄 白芍药 柴胡 甘草

(38)散风除湿活血汤《中医眼科临床实践》

羌活 独活 防风 前胡 当归 川芎 赤芍药 红花 鸡血藤 忍冬藤 苍术 白术 枳壳 甘草

(39)新制柴连汤《眼科纂要》

柴胡 川黄连 黄芩 赤芍药 蔓荆子 栀子 龙胆草 木通 甘草 荆芥 防风

(40)龙胆泻肝汤(李东垣方)

龙胆草 柴胡 泽泻 车前子 木通 生地黄 当归尾 栀子 黄芩 甘草

(41)托里消毒散《医宗金鉴》

黄芪 皂角刺 金银花 甘草 桔梗 白芷 川芎 当归 白芍 白术 茯苓 人参

(42)羌活胜风汤《原机启微》

柴胡 荆芥 防风 羌活 独活 薄荷 川芎 白芷 白术 甘草 枳壳 黄芩 桔梗 前胡

(43)知柏地黄汤《医宗金鉴》

知母 黄柏 熟地黄 山萸肉 淮山药 茯苓 泽泻 丹皮

(44)桑菊饮《温病条辨》

桑叶 菊花 苦杏仁 连翘 桔梗 薄荷 生甘草 芦根

(45)银花解毒汤《庞氏经验方》

银花 蒲公英 炙桑皮 花粉 黄芩 龙胆草 大黄 蔓荆子 枳壳

(46)大补阴丸《丹溪心法》

黄柏(盐炒) 知母(盐炒) 熟地 龟板

(47)香贝养荣汤《医宗金鉴》

白术 人参 茯苓 陈皮 熟地黄 川芎 当归 贝母 香附 白芍 桔梗 甘草 大枣 生姜

(48)参苓白术散《和剂局方》

党参　茯苓　白术　扁豆　陈皮　山药　炙甘草　莲子肉　薏苡仁　桔梗　缩砂仁

(49)肥儿丸《医宗金鉴》
人参　白术　茯苓　黄连　胡黄连　使君子　神曲　炒麦芽　炒山楂　炙甘草　芦荟

(50)附子理中汤《阎氏小儿方论》
附子　白术　干姜　党参　炙甘草

(51)抑阳酒连散《原机启微》
生地黄　独活　黄柏　防风　知母　蔓荆子　前胡　羌活　白芷　生甘草　黄芩　寒水石　栀子　黄连　防己

(52)杞菊地黄汤《医宗金鉴》
熟地黄　山萸肉　炒山药　泽泻　茯苓　丹皮　枸杞　菊花

(53)益气聪明汤《脾胃论》
蔓荆子　黄芪　人参　黄柏　白芍药　炙甘草　升麻　葛根

(54)甘露饮《和剂局方》
生地黄　熟地黄　石斛　天门冬　麦门冬　黄芩　茵陈　枳壳　甘草　枇杷叶

(55)除风益损汤《审视瑶函》
当归　白芍　熟地黄　川芎　藁本　前胡　防风

(56)明目地黄汤《审视瑶函》
熟地黄　山萸肉　炒山药　泽泻　茯神　生地黄　柴胡　当归　五味

子 丹皮

(57)丹栀逍遥散《和剂局方》

柴胡 当归 白芍药 茯苓 白术 甘草 薄荷 生姜 丹皮 栀子

(58)绿风羚羊饮《医宗金鉴》

黑玄参 防风 茯苓 知母 黄芩 细辛 桔梗 羚羊角 车前子 大黄

(59)半夏羚羊角散《审视瑶函》

羚羊角 薄荷 羌活 半夏 白菊花 川乌 川芎 防风 车前子 细辛

(60)羚羊钩藤饮《通俗伤寒论》

羚羊角粉 钩藤 桑叶 菊花 生地黄 白芍 甘草 贝母 竹茹 茯神

(61)羚羊角散《普济方》

羚羊角屑 茯神 车前子 甘菊花 决明子 羌活 防风 赤芍 蔓荆子 黄芩 升麻 山栀子 麦门冬 甘草 柴胡 枳壳

(62)通窍活血汤《医林改错》

赤芍 川芎 桃仁 红花 红枣 鲜姜 老葱 麝香

(63)涤痰汤《济生方》

半夏 橘红 白茯苓 甘草 生姜 胆南星 枳实 人参 菖蒲 竹茹 大枣

(64)天麻钩藤饮《杂病证治新义》

天麻　钩藤　生决明　山栀子　黄芩　川牛膝　杜仲　益母草　桑寄生　夜交藤　茯神

(65)加减驻景丸《中医眼科六经法要》

菟丝子　褚实子　茺蔚子　枸杞子　车前子　木瓜　寒水石　紫河车粉　生三七　五味子

(66)人参养荣汤《和剂局方》

人参　白茯苓　白术　炙甘草　当归　熟地黄　白芍药　肉桂　黄芪　远志　陈皮　五味子　生姜　大枣

(67)右归丸《景岳全书》

熟地黄　山萸肉　炒山药　枸杞　杜仲　当归　肉桂　附子　菟丝子　鹿角胶

(68)八珍汤《正体类要》

人参　白术　白茯苓　当归　川芎　白芍药　熟地黄　甘草

(69)宁血汤(经验方)

仙鹤草　旱莲草　生地黄　栀子炭　白芍　白芨　白蔹　侧柏叶　阿胶　白茅根

(70)祛淤汤《中医眼科学》

川芎　当归尾　桃仁　赤芍　生地黄　旱莲草　泽兰　丹参　仙鹤草　郁金

(71)仙方活命饮《校注妇人良方》

白芷　贝母　防风　赤芍药　当归尾　甘草节　皂角刺　天花粉　乳香　没药　金银花　陈皮　穿山甲

(72)泻脑汤《审视瑶函》

防风　车前子　木通　茺蔚子　茯苓　大黄　玄参　玄明粉　桔梗　黄芩

(73)通幽汤《兰室秘藏》

炙甘草　红花　生地黄　熟地黄　升麻　桃仁　当归

(74)小续命汤《千金方》

麻黄　防己　人参　黄芩　桂心　甘草　芍药　川芎　杏仁　附子　防风　生姜

(75)六君子汤《医学正传》

人参　白术　茯苓　甘草　陈皮　半夏　生姜　大枣

(76)正容汤《审视瑶函》

羌活　白附子　防风　秦艽　胆南星　僵蚕　法半夏　木瓜　松节　甘草　生姜

(77)补阳还五汤《医林改错》

黄芪　当归尾　赤芍　地龙　川芎　桃仁　红花

(78)桃红四物汤《医宗金鉴》

桃仁　红花　当归　生地黄　赤芍药　川芎

(79)通血丸《证治准绳》

生地黄　赤芍药　甘草　川芎　防风　荆芥　当归

(80)十灰散《十药神书》

大蓟　小蓟　荷叶　侧柏叶　白茅根　茜草根　山栀子　大黄　丹皮　棕榈皮

(81)犀角地黄汤《备急千金要方》
犀角　生地黄　芍药　丹皮

(82)归脾汤《济生方》
白术　茯苓　黄芪　人参　龙眼肉　酸枣仁　木香　甘草　当归　远志

(83)逍遥散《和剂局方》
柴胡　当归　白芍药　白术　茯苓　炙甘草　薄荷　生姜

(84)如意金黄散《医宗金鉴》
大黄　黄柏　姜黄　白芷各2.5千克　胆南星　陈皮　苍术　厚朴甘草各1千克　天花粉5千克　共为细末

(85)敷烂弦眼方《审视瑶函》
炉甘石30克(煅飞过)　飞丹(飞朱砂)15克　枯矾7.5克　明朱砂研细3克　铜绿6克　共为一处　研极细为度

(86)紫金锭《片玉心书》
雄黄　朱砂　麝香　五倍子　红芽大戟去芦　山慈菇洗去皮毛　续随子肉去油　共研细末，用糯米粉打糊作锭，每锭重0.03克。

(87)外障眼药水(经验方)
黄连15克　风化硝9克　硼砂0.6克　西红花1.5克　清水1500克煎30分钟，过滤后加防腐剂。

(88)黄连西瓜霜眼液(经验方)

黄连素 0.5 克　西瓜霜 5.0 克　月石 0.2 克　硝苯汞 0.002 克　蒸馏水 100ml。

(89)10%千里光眼液《医院制剂》

千里光全草 10 克，乙醇浸泡，浓缩脱色等，最后加蒸馏水至 100 毫升。

(90)1%黄芩素眼液《中医眼科学》

黄芩素结晶 1 克，加蒸馏水 100 毫升，加氢氧化钠调整 pH 为 7 左右，再加 0.9%氯化纳及 0.001%硝基苯汞为防腐剂。

(91)犀黄散《中医眼科学讲义》

西月石粉 15 克　冰片 9 克　麝香 0.9 克　犀黄 1.2 克　共研极细末。

(92)春雪膏《普济方》

冰片 3 克　蕤仁去壳 6 克　麝香 1.5 克　研极细末用蜜相合成膏。

(93)五胆膏《医宗金鉴》

猪胆汁　黄牛胆汁　羊胆汁　鲤鱼胆汁　熊胆　胡黄连末　川黄连末　青皮末各 7.5 克　白蜜 60 克　将诸药和匀，入瓷瓶封牢，做饭上蒸，待饭熟为度。

(94)10%黄连液《眼科临证录》

黄连 10 克　水煎沸，过滤后配成 100 毫升药液，加防腐剂高压消毒。

(95)银黄注射液《医院制剂》

金银花提取物 12.5 克　黄芩提取物 20 克　苯甲醇 10ml　注射用水适量　共制成 1000 毫升　过滤灌封　消毒灭菌

(96)10%穿心莲眼液《中医眼科学》

穿心莲浸膏粉 3 克　加蒸馏水 100 毫升，调整 pH 值，加防腐剂。

(97)三黄眼液《中医眼科学》

川黄连 6 克　黄芩 6 克　黄柏 6 克　加水煮沸两次，过滤浓缩至 200ml，加适量月石，调整 pH 值，过滤后消毒备用。

(98)退云散《眼科临症录》

冰香散 10 克　制甘石 60 克为甲组药　黄柏　黄芩　黄连　防风　蝉蜕　白芷　羌活　薄荷　川芎　白菊花　荆芥　当归　大黄　赤芍　连翘　木贼草各 3 克为乙组药　海螵蛸 6 克　荸荠粉 9 克　冰片 7.5 克　西黄 0.6 克　珠粉 1.2 克　熊胆 0.6 克　淡硇砂 0.3 克　朱砂 3 克　蕤仁霜 3 克　麝香 0.75 克为丙组药，先将乙组药加水煮沸过滤，再加甲组药，日光晒干，研磨极精细后加丙组药，再研磨极细，密封备用。

(99)2%槟榔碱滴眼液《中医眼科学》

(100)1%丁公藤碱滴眼液《中医眼科学》

(101)羚翘解毒丸《全国中成药处方集》

金银花　连翘　桔梗　牛蒡子　薄荷　竹叶　荆芥穗　甘草　淡豆豉　羚羊角

(102)黄连上清丸《全国中成药处方集》

黄连　黄芩　黄柏　栀子　菊花　当归　桔梗　葛根　薄荷　玄参　天花粉　川芎　姜黄　连翘　大黄

(103)牛黄解毒片《幼科证治准绳》

牛黄　甘草　金银花　草河车

(104)人参健脾丸《杂病证治类方》

　　白术　白茯苓　人参　神曲　陈皮　砂仁　麦芽　山楂　山药　肉豆蔻　木香　黄连　甘草

(105)十全大补丸《和剂局方》

人参　白术　炙甘草　当归　川芎　白芍药　熟地　黄芪　肉桂

(106)牛黄清心丸《痘疹世医心法》

牛黄　朱砂　生黄连　黄芩　栀子　郁金

(107)养阴清肺丸《全国中成药处方集》

生地　玄参　浙贝母　薄荷　麦冬　丹皮　生白芍　甘草

(108)六味地黄丸《小儿药证直诀》

熟地黄　山萸肉　干山药　泽泻　茯苓　丹皮

(109)石斛夜光丸《原机启微》

天门冬　麦门冬　人参　茯苓　熟地黄　生地黄　牛膝　杏仁　枸杞子　草决明　川芎　犀角　白蒺藜　羚羊角　枳壳　石斛　五味子　青葙子　甘草　防风　肉苁蓉　川黄连　菊花　山药　菟丝子

(110)杞菊地黄丸：同杞菊地黄汤

(111)逍遥丸：同逍遥散

(112)龙胆泻肝丸：同龙胆泻肝汤

(113)知柏地黄丸: 同知柏地黄汤

(114)明目地黄丸: 同明目地黄汤

(115)补中益气丸: 同补中益气汤

(116)安神镇惊丸《明医杂著》
天竺黄　人参　茯神　南星姜制　酸枣仁(炒)　麦冬　当归　生地黄　赤芍　薄荷　木通　黄连　山栀　辰砂　牛黄　龙骨　青黛。

THE ENGLISH–CHINESE ENCYCLOPEDIA OF PRACTICAL TCM
(Booklist)
英汉实用中医药大全
(书目)

VOLUME	TITLE	书名
1	ESSENTIALS OF TRADITIONAL CHINESE MEDICINE	中医学基础
2	THE CHINESE MATERIA MEDICA	中药学
3	PHARMACOLOGY OF TRADITIONAL CHINESE MEDICAL FORMULAE	方剂学
4	SIMPLE AND PROVEN PRESCRIPTION	单验方
5	COMMONLY USED CHINESE PATENTMEDICINES	常用中成药
6	THERAPY OF ACUPUNCTURE AND MOXIBUSTION	针灸疗法
7	*TUINA* THERAPY	推拿疗法
8	MEDICAL *QIGONG*	医学气功
9	MAINTAINING YOUR HEALTH	自我保健
10	INTERNAL MEDICINE	内科学

11	SURGERY	外科学
12	GYNECOLOGY	妇科学
13	PEDIATRICS	儿科学
14	ORTHOPEDICS	骨伤科学
15	PROCTOLOGY	肛门直肠病学
16	DERMATOLOGY	皮肤病学
17	OPHTHALMOLOGY	眼科学
18	OTORHINOLARYNGOLOGY	耳鼻喉科学
19	EMERGENTOLOGY	急症学
20	NURSING	护理
21	CLINICAL DIALOGUE	临床会话